D0863634

DON'T VACCINATE BEFORE YOU EDUCATE

Mayer Eisenstein, M.D., J.D., M.P.H.

Don't Vaccinate Before You Educate
Mayer Eisenstein, M.D., J.D., M.P.H.

Published by CMI Press
http://www.homefirst.com

ISBN 0-9670444-2-1 $16.95

HOMEFIRST® HEALTH SERVICES VACCINE POLICY STATEMENT

The physicians of Homefirst® Health Services follow the guidelines of the American Academy of Pediatrics and the Illinois Department of Public Health with regard to childhood vaccinations. However, unlike many other physicians, we will be honored to serve your family if you decide to vaccinate your children with all, some or none of the vaccines.

TABLE OF CONTENTS

FOREWORD

Don't Vaccinate Before You Educate is the sum collection of my 30 years as a father, grandfather, practicing physician, public health doctor and now also as an attorney. Many of the items come from discussions at my monthly vaccine seminars (see schedule at www.homefirst.com). This book is not meant to convince you to vaccinate or not vaccinate your children but to open your eyes to the ongoing debate.

> Education as defined by Webster's College Dictionary:
>
> To impart knowledge to; provide with information; *to educate consumers*

To educate means to widen one's horizons. I hope that this book will be educational with regard to the vaccine issues and inspire you to become more educated with regard to the risk vs. benefits of vaccine programs.

I have included just a few of the many pro and con scientific vaccine studies. Many more can be obtained by going on the internet to the multiple vaccine sites as well as to the on-line versions of some of the most prestigious medical journals (BMJ, AMA, Pediatrics, Lancet, Journal of Disease of Children).

In Chapter II I have included the opening statements from United States Congressman Dan Burton's Committee on Conflicts of Interest in Vaccine Development. This Committee pointed out the close association and financial ties of vaccine researchers and the vaccine manufacturers. I then bring you a pro vaccine editorial from the *Journal of the American Medical Association* written by Dr. Edwards whose funding comes in part from the major drug companies which sell vaccines. This serious problem lends questions of credibility to vaccine development and ongoing vaccine research.

I then bring you chapters on chicken pox, hepatitis B and flu vaccine which come from my previous book *Safer Medicine*. It is interesting that when *Safer Medicine* was written in August of 2000, just hepatitis B vaccine was mandated in Illinois. Just recently (April 2002) chicken pox vaccine has become mandated in Illinois. I believe that in the near future the flu vaccine will also be included on the ever growing list of mandated in Illinois and most states. The credibility of the vaccine programs lie not with their strongest links (i.e. alleged eradication of smallpox and the soon to be alleged eradication of polio), but with their weakest links (mandates for hepatitis B, chicken pox and flu vaccines, as well as the negative effects experienced i.e. non-hodgkin lymphoma from SV40 - see page 42 - mercury toxicity, autism, etc.).

The issue of confidentiality in medicine, which I discussed in Chapter VI, is a topic I researched while in law school. I came to the conclusion that doctors, unlike attorneys and clergy, no longer honor confidential statements made to them. This is in direct violation of the Hippocratic Oath.

In Chapter VII, I discuss vaccine law, the different forms of objections to vaccines (medical, religious and philosophical). In Appendix E I bring you the legal elements of "an Illinois Religious Exemption Letter to Childhood Vaccines". This letter is meant to be utilized by families in creating their own sincere personal letter of religious belief against vaccines in order to be in compliance with the law.

Appendix F "Questions and Answers" are from the most commonly asked questions at the Homefirst® Vaccine Seminars.

I hope this book leads you to do more research as well as think about your religious and spiritual convictions. Thank you for giving me the opportunity to serve so many families. God bless.

Mayer Eisenstein, M.D., J.D., M.P.H.

INTRODUCTION

In 1970, Robert Mendelsohn, M.D., my pediatrics professor and godfather to my six children, believed in the value of vaccinations. After 1970, he began to question the general value of mass immunization. In 1971, he stopped administering the Measles, Mumps, Rubella Vaccine (MMR), by 1973, he gave up on the Diphtheria, Pertussis, Tetanus Vaccine (DPT) and by 1976 he gave up on the Oral Polio Vaccine (OPV). By 1989 Dr. Mendelsohn no longer recommended any vaccines.

More and more families, after carefully weighing the evidence, are deciding not to vaccinate their children. My goal is for you to make an educated decision.

I want to raise doubt in your mind as to the safety, efficacy and moral issues of vaccines. My goal is for you to do further research into all of the vaccines, use libraries, bookstores, our internet web site (homefirst.com) and ask questions. Only after fully weighing the evidence can you make an informed decision. An informed consumer is a wise consumer. This journey is a beginning of better understanding the issues surrounding childhood vaccinations.

CECRECRE

The following information was learned over the many years that I was a student of Dr. Mendelsohn. While a practicing physician, I was honored to be with Dr. Mendelsohn when he gave lectures to medical societies and university classes on his philosophy of medicine. We discussed these issues many times over the years. He later compiled much of this information into his books *Confessions of a Medical Heretic* and *How To Raise A Healthy Child... In Spite of Your Doctor.*

IMMUNIZATION AGAINST DISEASE: A MEDICAL TIME BOMB?

The greatest threat of childhood diseases lies in the dangerous and ineffectual efforts made to prevent them through mass immunization.

...Doctors, not politicians, have successfully lobbied for laws that force parents to immunize their children as a prerequisite for admission to school.

...They [doctors] should be nervous, because in a recent Chicago case a child damaged by a pertussis inoculation received a $5.5 million settlement award. If your doctor is in that state of mind, exploit his fear, because your child's health is at stake.

Although I administered them myself during my early years of practice, I have become a steadfast opponent of mass inoculations because of the myriad hazards they present....

Here Is the Core of My Concern

1.   There is no convincing scientific evidence that mass inoculations can be credited with eliminating any childhood disease....

2.   It is commonly believed that the Salk vaccine was responsible for halting the polio epidemics that plagued American children in the 1940's and 1950's. If so, why did the epidemics also end in Europe, where polio vaccine was not so extensively used?...

3.   There are significant risks associated with every immunization and numerous contraindications that may make it dangerous for the shots to be given to your child....

4.   While the myriad short-term hazards of most immunizations are known (but rarely explained), no one knows the long-term consequences of injecting foreign proteins into the body of your child. Even more shocking is the fact that no one is making any structured effort to find out.

5.   There is a growing suspicion that immunization against relatively harmless childhood diseases may be responsible for the dramatic increase in autoimmune diseases since mass inoculations were introduced. These are fearful diseases such as cancer, leukemia, rheumatoid arthritis, multiple sclerosis, Lou Gehrig's disease, lupus and the Guillain-Barré syndrome....

...As a parent, only you can decide whether to reject immunizations or risk accepting them for your child. Let me urge you, though—before your child is immunized—to arm yourself with the facts about the potential risks and benefits and demand that your pediatrician defend the immunizations that he recommends.

  CBCRCBCR

WHAT'S IN A VACCINE?

Vaccines contain many ingredients of which the public is not aware. These are just some of the ingredients used to make a vaccine:

* Ethylene glycol - antifreeze

* Phenol - also known as carbolic acid. This is used as a disinfectant, dye.

* Formaldehyde - a known cancer causing agent

*Aluminum - which is associated with Alzheimer's disease and seizures also cancer producing in laboratory mice. It is used as an additive to promote antibody response.

* Thimerosal - a mercury disinfectant/preservative. It can result in brain injury and autoimmune disease.

* Neomycin, Streptomycin - antibiotics which have caused allergic reaction in some people.

These vaccines are also grown on and strained thru animal or human tissue such as monkey kidney tissue, chicken embryo, embryonic guinea pig cells, calf serum, human diploid cells (the dissected organs of aborted fetuses as in the case of rubella, hepatitis A, and chicken pox vaccines)

The problem with using animal cells is that during serial passage of the virus thru the animal cells, animal RNA and DNA can be transferred from one host to another. Undetected animal viruses may slip past quality control testing procedures, as happened during the years 1955 thru 1961. The polio vaccine, which was grown on the kidney of the Green African monkey (simian), was contaminated with SV40 (simian virus

#40 - the 40th discovered) which differs from the other 39 because it has oncogenic (cancer causing) properties. What other viruses could be slipping by from animal tissue, administered through vaccinations, that we don't know of?

Chapter I

CHILDHOOD VACCINE
PROS AND CONS

All vaccine programs carry risk and benefit. Therefore, the goal should not only be the prevention of a specific disease by vaccination, the benefits must *outweigh* any potential long term negative side effects. For example, as a public health measure, if children do not get polio because of the polio vaccine but later die of a cancer caused by the SV40 virus received as a contaminant in the vaccine, the risk *may* outweigh the benefits.

Vaccine proponents claim that the benefits of childhood vaccination are undeniable. However, at the same time vaccine opponents point out that the incidents of autism, diabetes, and other chronic immune and neurological dysfunction in children have increased dramatically in the last 30 years. This points out the difficulty in making an informed decision to vaccinate or not to vaccinate if your only basis is the scientific literature. Here are medical studies both pro and con.

PROS
SCIENTIFIC ARTICLES
DOCUMENTING THE BENEFITS
OF CHILDHOOD VACCINATIONS

In the *New England Journal of Medicine* 345:656-661 2001, Davis, L. Robert, M.D., M.P.H., et al., studied "The Risk of Seizures after Receipt of Whole Cell Pertussis or Measles, Mumps, and Rubella Vaccine" and had the following results...

> "Receipt of DPT vaccine was associated with an increased risk of febrile seizures only on the day of vaccination..... Receipt of MMR vaccine was associated with an increased risk of febrile seizures 8-14 days after vaccination.... As compared with other children with febrile seizures that were not associated with vaccination, **the children who had febrile seizures after vaccination were not found to be at higher risk for subsequent seizures or neurodevelopmental disabilities**." He concluded "There are significantly elevated risks of febrile seizures after receipt of DTP vaccine or MMR vaccine, but these risks do not appear to be associated with any long term adverse consequences."

Dr. Davis goes on to say..

> While it's possible to prevent febrile
> seizures by giving kids Tylenol, he advises
> parents to talk to their doctor beforehand.
> "No medication is risk-free," he adds. "We
> don't want to promote the indiscriminate
> use of Tylenol."

*****

M.E. Comments

*When doctors believe that Tylenol may be more risky
than childhood vaccines, we have serious problems.
"We don't want to promote the indiscriminate use of
Tylenol" Dr. Davis says. What about the indiscriminate
use of vaccines? When the paradigm is "vaccinate
before you educate" no amount of risk will stop
physicians from vaccinating.*

At the **37th Annual Meeting of the Infectious Disease Society of America** 1999, lead researcher David W. Scheifele concluded,

> The newest whooping cough vaccine has a tenfold reduction in fever and significant amount of reduction of soreness at the injection site.... In terms of seizures and rag doll reactions, again the frequency is reduced five to ten fold... In terms of effectiveness the new vaccines (DtaP) are probably as good or probably even better.

*****

M.E. Comments

Doctors do not let go of one treatment until they find a more dangerous one to replace it. Just give them time with the new DtaP vaccine and they will find more and more problems. At least they now admit the old vaccines had problems.

In the *Archives of Disease of Children* 2001;84:227-229 (March), Miller, E, et al., studied "Idiopathic thrombocytopenic purpura and MMR vaccine" and concluded that...

> *A CAUSAL ASSOCIATION BETWEEN MEASLES* mumps-rubella (MMR) vaccine and idiopathic thrombocytopenic purpura (ITP) was confirmed using immunisation/hospital admission record linkage. The absolute risk within six weeks of immunisation was 1 in 22 300 doses, with two of every three cases occurring in the six week post-immunisation period being caused by MMR. Children with ITP before MMR had no vaccine associated recurrences.

Dr. Miller goes on to say...

> Our study confirms a causal association between MMR vaccine and ITP. The best estimate of absolute risk within six weeks of MMR is 1 in 22 300 doses, with two of every three cases being vaccine attributable. This is similar to previous

estimates, but is considerably less than ITP after natural measles (common), rubella (about 1 in 3000 cases), or mumps (rare). Over 70% of cases of ITP follow virus infections.

The component of MMR vaccine which is responsible for vaccine associated ITP is uncertain, but both the measles and rubella components are likely candidates.

Our results provide clear evidence that children with a history of ITP prior to the first dose of MMR vaccine are not at increased risk of a vaccine associated episode. Moreover the vaccine associated cases tended to be milder than others and not associated with a subsequent recurrence. A history of ITP should not therefore be considered a contraindication to MMR immunisation. Although there have been occasional case reports of children with ITP after repeated doses of MMR or measles containing vaccines, there has been no systematic study of the outcome where a second dose of MMR is given to a child who developed

ITP after the first dose. We plan to investigate this using record linkage methodology following the introduction of the second dose of MMR in 1996. The recommendation of the American Committee of Immunization Practices does not absolutely contraindicate a second dose of MMR vaccine in children who develop ITP after the first dose, although it suggests that under these circumstances serological evidence of measles immunity may be sought as an alternative to repeat MMR immunisation. The logic of this recommendation is unclear. If, as seems likely, vaccine associated ITP is usually related to susceptibility to the measles or other component of the vaccine with consequent viral replication, then seropositive children should be without risk while reimmunisation of those who are seronegative would be recommended on the grounds of protection against the wild virus infection. Information on the outcome of reimmunisation in children with a history of vaccine associated ITP is required in order to formulate a rational policy.

M.E. COMMENTS

I thought the goal of vaccine programs was to lower risk in the population. If you continue to experience the risk of ITP (as explained above) with the MMR vaccine, you better make sure that other risks associated with the MMR vaccine do not tip the risk vs. benefit ratio away from the benefit.

In *The Lancet* Volume 358, Number 9289 13 October 2001, Simonsen, L., et al., studied "Effect of rotavirus vaccination programme on trends in admission of infants to hospital for intussusception" and found that...

Studies have reported a temporal association between a first dose of rotavirus vaccine (Rotashield) and infant intussusception. We investigated the effect of Rotashield vaccination use on intussusception admissions in ten US states.

We analysed electronic databases containing 100% hospital discharge records for 1993-99 from ten US states, where an estimated 28% of the birth cohort had received Rotashield (based on manufacturer's net sales data). We examined records of infants admitted to hospital (<365 days old) with any mention of intussusception (International Classification of Diseases, ninth revision, clinical modification code 560·0). Excess admissions for intussusception during the period of Rotashield availability (October

1998 to June 1999) were estimated by direct comparison with the corresponding period of October 1997 to June 1998 (before Rotashield was available) and with adjustment for secular trends during 1993-98 by Poisson regression.

Hospital admission for intussusception among infants younger than 365 days of age during the Rotashield period compared with previously was 4% lower (10 cases) by direct comparison and 10% lower (27 cases) by trend comparison, corresponding to a negative population attributable risk. Among infants aged 45-210 days (target age range for a first Rotashield dose), we estimated an increase in intussusception admissions of 1% (one excess admission) by direct comparison and 4% (4-6 excess admissions) by trend comparison, corresponding to a population attributable risk range of one excess admission in 66 000-302 000.

Simonson, et. al., interpreted the results to mean...

We found no evidence of increased infant intussusception admissions during the period of Rotashield availability. The total intussusception admission risk attributable to Rotashield was substantially lower than previous estimates based on studies focusing on the immediate postvaccination weeks.

Lancet 2001; 358: 1224-29

In a Special Article in *PEDIATRICS* Vol. 109 No. 1 January 2002, pp. 124-129 Offit, Paul A., M.D., et al.,"Addressing Parents Concerns: Do Multiple Vaccines Overwhelm or Weaken the Infant's Immune System?" found that...

>Recent surveys found that an increasing number of parents are concerned that infants receive too many vaccines. Implicit in this concern is that the infant"s immune system is inadequately developed to handle vaccines safely or that multiple vaccines may overwhelm the immune system. In this review, we will examine the following: 1) the ontogeny of the active immune response and the ability of neonates and young infants to respond to vaccines; 2) the theoretic capacity of an infant's immune system; 3) data that demonstrate that mild or moderate illness does not interfere with an infant"s ability to generate protective immune responses to vaccines; 4) how infants respond to vaccines given in combination compared with the same vaccines given separately; 5) data showing that vaccinated children are not more likely to develop infections with

other pathogens than unvaccinated children; and 6) the fact that infants actually encounter fewer antigens in vaccines today than they did 40 or 100 years ago.

DO VACCINES "OVERWHELM" THE IMMUNE SYSTEM?

Infants Have the Capacity to Respond to an Enormous Number of Antigens Studies on the diversity of antigen receptors indicate that the immune system has the capacity to respond to extremely large numbers of antigens. Current data suggest that the theoretical capacity determined by diversity of antibody variable gene regions would allow for as many as 10,000 different antibody specificities. But this prediction is limited by the number of circulating B cells and the likely redundancy of antibodies generated by an individual.

A more practical way to determine the diversity of the immune response would be to estimate the number of vaccines to which a child could respond at one time.... [The immune system] would have the theoretical capacity to respond to about 10,000 vaccines at any one time.

SUMMARY

Current studies do not support the hypothesis that multiple vaccines overwhelm, weaken, or "use up" the immune system. On the contrary, young infants have an enormous capacity to respond to multiple vaccines, as well as to the many other challenges present in the environment. By providing protection against a number of bacterial and viral pathogens, vaccines prevent the "weakening" of the immune system and consequent secondary bacterial infections occasionally caused by natural infection.

M.E. Comments

For a revelation as to who Dr. Paul Offit is see page 57. He certainly is not an unbiased physician in the vaccine debate. In his informative free weekly health newsletter Dr. Joe Mercola comments on Dr. Offit's article Issue 310 March 27, 2002. To subscribe to this outstanding free newsletter go to www.mercola.com.

The concept that 10,000 antigens could theoretically be deposited uneventfully into the blood stream of either an infant or an adult defies logic and is a blatant

disregard for mechanisms of human physiology.

Once again, a "ground breaking" medical study has drawn media attention by posting conclusions that are not supported by facts. Stating that an infant has a large capacity to respond to antigens, i.e. create an antibody response, does nothing to allay reasonable fears and doubts by investigative parents.

Any "thinking doctor" should recognize this "study" for what it is: another opportunity to spread the mantra of "safe and effective" vaccines. Perhaps in this way we won't question the more than 200 vaccines that are currently in development or resist the more than 20 that are anticipated to become part of the childhood vaccination schedule by 2010.

A "thinking parent" might conclude that, "if the immune system is that strong, why do we need to vaccinate at all?

In a Review Article *in PEDIATRICS* Vol. 107 No. 5 May 2001, pp. 1147-1154 "An Assessment of Thimerosal Use in Childhood Vaccines" Ball, Leslie K., et al., stated

> On July 7, 1999, the American Academy of Pediatrics and the US Public Health Service issued a joint statement calling for removal of thimerosal, a mercury-containing preservative, from vaccines. This action was prompted in part by a risk assessment from the Food and Drug Administration that is presented here.

Results.

> Delayed-type hypersensitivity reactions from thimerosal exposure are well-recognized. Identified acute toxicity from inadvertent high-dose exposure to thimerosal includes neurotoxicity and nephrotoxicity. Limited data on toxicity from low-dose exposures to ethylmercury are available, but toxicity may be similar to that of methylmercury. Chronic, low-dose methylmercury exposure may cause subtle neurologic abnormalities. Depending on the immunization schedule,

vaccine formulation, and infant weight, cumulative exposure of infants to mercury from thimerosal during the first 6 months of life may exceed EPA guidelines.

Conclusion.

Our review revealed no evidence of harm caused by doses of thimerosal in vaccines, except for local hypersensitivity reactions. However, some infants may be exposed to cumulative levels of mercury during the first 6 months of life that exceed EPA recommendations. Exposure of infants to mercury in vaccines can be reduced or eliminated by using products formulated without thimerosal as a preservative.

M.E. Comments

Would you call this doubletalk? There is no harm from thimerosal in any dose, just be careful about the accumulation. If there is no harm, why was the thimerosal removed from the vaccines?

In the *BMJ* 2002;324:393-396 (16 February)
"Measles, mumps, and rubella vaccination and bowel
problems or developmental regression in children with
autism: population study" Taylor, Brent , et al.,
reported the following findings...

Objectives:

> To investigate whether measles, mumps,
> and rubella (MMR) vaccination is
> associated with bowel problems and
> developmental regression in children with
> autism, looking for evidence of a "new
> variant" form of autism.

Results:

> The proportion of children with
> developmental regression (25% overall) or
> bowel symptoms (17%) did not change
> significantly (P value for trend 0.50 and
> 0.47, respectively) during the 20 years
> from 1979, a period which included the
> introduction of MMR vaccination in
> October 1988. No significant difference
> was found in rates of bowel problems or
> regression in children who received the
> MMR vaccine before their parents became

concerned about their development (where MMR might have caused or triggered the autism with regression or bowel problem), compared with those who received it only after such concern and those who had not received the MMR vaccine. A possible association between non-specific bowel problems and regression in children with autism was seen but this was unrelated to MMR vaccination.

Conclusions:

These findings provide no support for an MMR associated "new variant" form of autism with developmental regression and bowel problems, and further evidence against involvement of MMR vaccine in the initiation of autism.

In *Family Practice News* Vol. 32;6:1 "Flu Vaccine Urged For Infants, Families" Senior Writer, Tucker, Miriam E. reported that...

> New guidelines "encourage" influenza vaccination of infants aged 6-23 months of age, with an eye toward a stronger universal recommendation in 1-3 years.

> The guidelines, approved at a meeting of the Centers for Disease Control and Prevention's Advisory Committee on Immunization Practices, also recommend flu vaccine for all household contacts—adults and children—of infants up to 24 months of age....

> Healthy children under 2 years of age have been added to the list of individuals known to be at high risk of influenza complications.

M.E. Comments
I predict that it will be a short while before the flu vaccine will become mandated for children. This is in keeping with the current medical paradigm "Vaccinate before you educate."

CONS
SCIENTIFIC ARTICLES
DOCUMENTING THE DETRIMENT
OF CHILDHOOD VACCINATIONS

In the *New England Journal of Medicine* Volume 344:564-572 February 22, 2001 Number 8 "Intussusception among Infants Given an Oral Rotavirus Vaccine" Murphy, Trudy V. M.D., et al., reported...

Background

> Intussusception is a form of intestinal obstruction in which a segment of the bowel prolapses into a more distal segment. Our investigation began on May 27, 1999, after nine cases of infants who had intussusception after receiving the tetravalent rhesus—human reassortant rotavirus vaccine (RRV-TV) were reported to the Vaccine Adverse Event Reporting System

Results

> Data were analyzed for 429 infants with intussusception and 1763 matched controls in a case—control analysis as well as for 432 infants with intussusception in a case-series analysis. Seventy-four of the 429 infants with intussusception (17.2 percent) and 226 of the 1763 controls (12.8 percent) had received RRV-TV

(P=0.02). An increased risk of intussusception 3 to 14 days after the first dose of RRV-TV was found in the case—control analysis (adjusted odds ratio, 21.7; 95 percent confidence interval, 9.6 to 48.9). In the case-series analysis, the incidence-rate ratio was 29.4 (95 percent confidence interval, 16.1 to 53.6) for days 3 through 14 after a first dose. There was also an increase in the risk of intussusception after the second dose of the vaccine, but it was smaller than the increase in risk after the first dose. Assuming full implementation of a national program of vaccination with RRV-TV, we estimated that 1 case of intussusception attributable to the vaccine would occur for every 4670 to 9474 infants vaccinated.

Conclusions

The strong association between vaccination with RRV-TV (Rotavirus Vaccine) and intussusception among otherwise healthy infants supports the existence of a causal relation. Rotavirus vaccines with an improved safety profile are urgently needed.

M.E. Comments

What is one to believe? Is there or is there not a strong association with intussusception and Rotavirus vaccine? This very issue is one of the reasons why it is so difficult on scientific grounds to decide if you should or should not vaccinate.

In *The Journal of Infectious Diseases* 2001;184:1293-1299 "Magnitude of Interference after Diphtheria-Tetanus ToxoidsAcellular Pertussis/*Haemophilus influenzae* Type b Capsular PolysaccharideTetanus Vaccination Is Related to the Number of Doses Administered" Daum, Robert S. M.D., et al., reported...

We compared the antibody response to *Haemophilus influenzae* type b capsular polysaccharide (PRP) after 1, 2, or 3 doses of DTaP vaccine combined with a PRP-T vaccine, followed by separate injections of DTaP and PRP-T vaccines for the last 1 or 2 doses. Healthy infants were recruited from pediatric practices and were immunized according to recommended schedules. A significant decrease in the mean anti-PRP (from 5.25 to 2.68 g/mL) and antitetanus toxoid antibody responses (from 0.13 to 0.09 Eq/mL) was observed as the number of doses of the DTaP/PRP-T combination vaccine increased ($P < .02$ and $P = .01$, respectively). In contrast, the mean antidiphtheria toxoid antibody response increased with increasing numbers of DTaP/PRP-T doses ($P =$ .0001). The effects of interference were not eliminated by the completion of the primary series with 1 or 2 doses of the DTaP and PRP-T vaccines given separately.

M.E. Comments

This study reveals a weakened immune response to Haemophilus influenzae type b in children after immunization with a HIB/DTaP vaccine. This weakened immune response is directly correlated with the number of vaccine doses given. A far cry from the 10,000 vaccines that can be given at one time, like Dr. Offit would want you to believe (see page 15). Again, which study do we believe?

In *Lancet* 1998; 351: 637-41 February 1998 "Ileal-lymphoid-nodular hyperplasia, non-specific colitis, and pervasive developmental disorder in children", Wakefield, A J, M.D., reports the following:

Background
> We investigated a consecutive series of children with chronic enterocolitis and regressive developmental disorder.

Findings
> **Onset of behavioural symptoms was associated, by the parents, with measles, mumps, and rubella vaccination in eight of the 12 children, with measles** infection in one child, and otitis media in another. All 12 children had intestinal abnormalities, ranging from lymphoid nodular hyperplasia to aphthoid ulceration. Histology showed patchy chronic inflammation in the colon in 11 children and reactive ileal lymphoid hyperplasia in seven, but no granulomas. Behavioural disorders included autism (nine), disintegrative psychosis (one), and possible postviral or vaccinal encephalitis

(two). There were no focal neurological abnormalities and MRI and EEG tests were normal. Abnormal laboratory results were significantly raised urinary methylmalonic acid compared with age-matched controls (p=0.003), low haemoglobin in four children, and a low serum IgA in four children.

Interpretation

We identified associated gastrointestinal disease and developmental regression in a group of previously normal children, which was generally associated in time with possible environmental triggers.

M.E. Comments

Dr. Wakefield says there are intestinal problems in autism associated with MMR vaccine. Other scientists say no. Who are you supposed to believe?

In *Lancet* Volume 351, Number 9106 21 March 1998, "Autism, inflammatory bowel disease, and MMR vaccine" author Wakefield, A J replies...

Author's reply

Sir--Our publication in *The Lancet* and the ensuing reaction throws into sharp relief the rift that can exist between clinical medicine and public health. Clinicians duties are to their patients, and the clinical researcher's obligation is to test hypotheses of disease pathogenesis on the basis of the story as it is presented to him by the patient or the patient's parent. Clearly, this is not the remit of public-health medicine. Accordingly, we have now investigated 48 children with developmental disorder in whom the parents said "my child has a problem with his/her bowels which I believe is related to their autism". Hitherto, this claim had been rejected by health professionals with little or no attempt to investigate the problem. The parents were right. They have helped us to identify a new inflammatory bowel disease that seems to be associated with their child's developmental disorder. This is a lesson in humility that, as doctors, we ignore at our peril. In many cases, the parents associated onset of behavioural symptoms in their child with MMR vaccine. Were we to ignore this because it challenged the public- health dogma on MMR vaccine safety? As they expound the virtues of MMR vaccine, public health officials would do well to reflect upon the fact that published pre-licensure studies of MMR vaccine safety have been restricted to 3 weeks. For three live viruses given in combination at a different dose, route, strain, and age, compared with the normal pattern of exposure of these viruses, 3 weeks seems woefully inadequate.

In citing pertussis as an example of how scare stories can damage health strategies, it is important to bear in mind that pertussis vaccine can be associated with neurological sequelae, albeit that the risks of the disease far outweigh those of vaccine. Recognition of this led to the passing of the Vaccine Damage Payments

Act in 1979. Until now, about 900 children have been awarded vaccine-damage payments, qualifying as 80% disabled. Had clinicians, in the conduct of their duty, not raised the issue of adverse neurological events with pertussis vaccine, shamefully, these children would have been put to one side, and there would have been no imperative for the production of a safer, acellular vaccine. Assumptions of vaccine safety, based upon inadequate safety trials and dogma contribute largely to confusion and public loss of confidence in vaccination. Public-health officials would do well to get their own house in order before attacking the position of either clinical researchers or *The Lancet* for what we perceive as our respective duties.

M.E. Comments

Dr. Mendelsohn used to say. "If you listen to a patient for five minutes they will tell you the problem and if you listen for another five minutes they will also give you the treatment". Dr. Wakefield personifies my late professor's philosophy. "The approach of the clinical scientists should reflect the first and most important lesson learnt as a medical student--to listen to the patient or the patient's parent, and they will tell you the answer." As a medical student Dr. Mendelsohn would tell us in the pediatric clinic - go see the patient in room 1. Don't take the chart with you, just listen. You will get all the answers. I have used the same philosophy for over 30 years with the same pleasure and gratification. It is exciting to see Dr. Wakefield recommending the same approach.

In *Lancet* 2001; 357: 381-84 "Proliferation-inducing viruses in non-permissive systems as possible causes of human cancers" Harald zur Hausen

Animal viruses, some of which are probably unable to replicate in human cells, could be transmitted to people where they may be linked to tumours currently not attributed to viruses. Several human virus types have oncogenic potential in animals. A potential risk for acquiring such infections by handling and preparation of animal products was analysed against the background of available epidemiological reports. Human tumours should be systematically assessed for proliferation-inducing viruses in non-permissive systems.

M.E. Comments
A scary article linking animal viruses (like SV40 see page 42)
with human cancers.

In *Lancet* 2002; 359: 817-23 "Association between simian virus 40 and non-Hodgkin lymphoma" Vilchez, Regis A, M.D., et. al.,

Background

> Non-Hodgkin lymphoma has increased in frequency over the past 30 years, and is a common cancer in HIV-1-infected patients. Although no definite risk factors have emerged, a viral cause has been postulated. Polyomaviruses are known to infect human beings and to induce tumours in laboratory animals. We aimed to identify which one of the three polyomaviruses able to infect human beings (simian virus 40 [SV40], JC virus, and BK virus) was associated with non-Hodgkin lymphoma.

Findings

> Polyomavirus T antigen sequences, all of which were SV40-specific, were detected in 64 (42%) of 154 non-Hodgkin lymphomas, none of 186 non-malignant lymphoid samples, and none of 54 control cancers. This difference was similar for HIV-1-infected patients and HIV-1-uninfected

patients alike. Few tumours were positive
for both SV40 and Epstein-Barr virus.
Human herpesvirus type 8 was not
detected. SV40 sequences were found
most frequently in diffuse large B-cell and
follicular-type lymphomas.

Interpretation

**SV40 is significantly associated with
some types of non-Hodgkin lymphoma.
These results add lymphomas to the
types of human cancers associated with
SV40.**

Discussion

This investigation showed that
polyomavirus SV40 T antigen DNA
sequences are significantly associated with
non-Hodgkin lymphoma in HIV-1-infected
and HIV-1-uninfected patients. This
finding sheds new light on the possible
genesis of an important group of
malignant disorders. The SV40 sequences
do not seem to be present simply because
non-Hodgkin lymphoma cells are readily
susceptible to viral infection; in that case,
EBV and SV40 should be found in similar

frequencies in non-Hodgkin lymphoma of HIV-1-infected and HIV-1-uninfected patients. The results also suggest that polyomavirus SV40 is not merely an opportunistic superinfection; if so, one would expect similar frequencies of SV40 detection in EBV-positive and EBV-negative non-Hodgkin lymphoma, and in other cancer samples (colon and breast) if those cell types wcre permissive to SV40 replication. The observation of minimal instances of coinfection with SV40 and EBV and the lack of detection of SV40 in non-malignant lymphoid samples and epithelial cancer control specimens suggest that SV40 might contribute to the development of those lymphomas in which it is present.

Polyomavirus SV40 has been associated with specific types of solid cancers in human beings, including brain tumours, osteosarcomas, and malignant mesotheliomas. These are the types of malignant disorders caused by the virus in laboratory animals--a finding that emphasises the predictive value of the animal studies. Recent reports provide persuasive evidence that the presence of polyomavirus SV40 is meaningful in the development of those human cancers. Immunohistochemical assays have detected the expression of T antigen in tumour cells, T-antigen protein complexed with p53 has been extracted from some cancer specimens, and microdissection of malignant mesothelioma samples followed by PCR assays detected SV40 DNA in tumour cells and not in adjacent non-malignant cells. When an antisense SV40 T antigen construct was introduced into SV40-DNA-positive malignant mesothelioma cell lines, the expression of T antigen was abrogated and growth was inhibited. ...

The major source of known human exposure to polyomavirus SV40 was immunisation with SV40-contaminated poliovaccines. Inactivated and live, attenuated forms of the poliovaccine were prepared in primary rhesus

monkey kidney cells, some of which were from animals naturally infected with SV40--a virus that was unknown at the time. Studies showed that residual infectious SV40 survived the vaccine inactivation treatments, and millions of people were inadvertently exposed to live SV40 from 1955 until early 1963. In the USA, vaccine lots received by about 20 states are estimated to have contained 0.75-0.97 mL contaminated vaccine per child, lots from about 15 states were thought to have contained 0.01-0.74 mL contaminated vaccine per child, and about 15 states were believed to have received lots that were free from SV40. Perhaps this distribution of contaminated vaccines influenced the differences in the rate of SV40-positive non-Hodgkin lymphoma that have been seen in recent studies. Seroepidemiological studies have shown the presence of SV40 neutralising antibodies in 16% of HIV-1-infected patients and 11% of HIV-1-uninfected individuals, some of whom were born after 1963 and could not have been exposed to

SV40-contaminated poliovaccines. Our study found that five patients with SV40-positive non-Hodgkin lymphoma were born after 1963--a finding similar to previous studies involving brain and bone cancers in which some patients with SV40-positive tumours had been born in recent decades. These observations suggest that polyomavirus SV40 might be causing infections in human beings long after the use of the contaminated vaccines. However, how SV40 is transmitted among humans, and the prevalence of infection, remain to be established.

In summary, our study suggests that polyomavirus SV40 is significantly associated with non-Hodgkin lymphoma in HIV-1-infected and HIV-1-uninfected patients and might have a role in the development of these haematological malignancies. Definition of a viral cofactor in the pathogenesis of these tumours could lead to new diagnostic, therapeutic, and preventative approaches.

In *Lancet* 2002; 359: 851-52 "Presence of simian virus 40 DNA sequences in human lymphomas" Shivapurkar, Narayan, M.D., et al.,

> Simian virus 40 (SV40)--a potent oncogenic virus–has been associated previously with some types of human tumours, but not with lymphomas. We examined human tumours for the presence of specific SV40 DNA sequences by PCR and Southern blotting. Viral sequences were present in 29 (43%) of 68 non-Hodgkin lymphomas, and in three (9%) of 31 of Hodgkin's lymphomas. Viral sequences were detected at low frequencies (about 5%) in 235 epithelial tumours of adult and paediatric origin, and were absent in 40 control tissues. **Our data suggest that SV40 might be a cofactor in the pathogenesis of non-Hodgkin lymphomas.**

M.E. Comments

The whole issue of SV40 contamination from polio vaccine is frightening. We are seeing more and more serious problems associated with SV40. Even scarier, some people who never received the contaminated vaccine which carried the SV40 virus, are dying from tumors associated with SV40. SV40 contamination became part of their genetic material transmitted to them from their parents who did receive the SV40 contaminated vaccine. How terrifying!!! In light of this vaccine side effect we have to be looking even into the next generation. This raises the issue will SV40 contamination of the polio vaccine cause more problems long term than polio ever did!!

41st Annual Interscience Conference on Antimicrobial Agents and Chemotherapy, Dr. Lee, et al., "Low varicella vaccine effectiveness identified at day care center"

> CHICAGO (Reuters Health) Dec 19, 2001 - New study findings indicate that, at least among one group of children, the varicella vaccine is much less effective than previously reported.
>
> Dr. Jane Seward, from the US Centers for Disease Control and Prevention in Atlanta, and colleagues reported Tuesday on their investigation of a recent outbreak of chickenpox at a New Hampshire day care center. They presented their findings here at the 41st Annual Interscience Conference on Antimicrobial Agents and Chemotherapy.
>
> The outbreak in 23 children began with a child who had been vaccinated, contradicting the belief that such "breakthrough" cases are not contagious, Dr. Seward noted. The child, a 4-year-old, was confirmed not to have developed

varicella infection from the vaccine, but probably developed it after exposure to a sibling with shingles.

Previous findings indicate that the vaccine's effectiveness ranges from 71% to 91%. In the current study, however, the effectiveness that was only about 40%. "Ours is the first study that has shown anything significantly below that level," co-author Dr. B. R. Lee of the CDC told Reuters Health.

Dr. Seward and Dr. Lee say they cannot yet explain why the vaccine was ineffective in this group of children. "We'd like to really understand what factors came together to produce it," Dr. Seward added. "We're not dismissing it."

M.E. COMMENTS
Why am I not shocked, as are Dr. Seward and Lee, that the Varicella Vaccine was ineffective in this group of children (effectiveness only about 40%)?

Vaccine, Vol. 18 (25) (2000) pp. 2775-2778 "Analysis of varicella vaccine breakthrough rates: implications for the effectiveness of immunisation programmes" Brisson, M., et al.,

Abstract

The objective of this study was to quantify key parameters describing varicella zoster virus (VZV) vaccine efficacy. To do so a mathematical model was developed to represent breakthrough cases as a function of time after vaccination in vaccine efficacy trials. Efficacy parameter sets were identified by fitting the predicted annual number of breakthrough infections with that observed in three clinical trials chosen to represent the plausible range of vaccine efficacy. **Results suggest that varicella vaccination seems to result in a high proportion of individuals who are initially totally protected (97% for the base-case). However, individuals lose full protection relatively rapidly (3% per year for the base-case). Once total protection has waned individuals have a high probability of developing a**

breakthrough infection if exposed to varicella (73% of the probability in unvaccinated susceptibles for the base-case). Results also highlight that vaccine efficacy parameters should be estimated concurrently to take into account dependencies between parameters.

M.E. COMMENTS

Let us assume that Varicella Vaccine is 97% effective and individuals lose full protection at the rate of 3% per year. Let us also assume that the vaccine is given on or before the fifth birthday. This would lead to a total lack of immunity by age 35, thus making a 35 year old adult susceptible to chicken pox, a relatively mild childhood disease, but a potentially very serious adult disease. See page 68.

References - Chapter I

Davis, L. Robert, M.D., M.P.H., et al., "The Risk of Seizures after Receipt of Whole Cell Pertussis or Measles, Mumps, and Rubella Vaccine", *New England Journal of Medicine* 345:656-661 2001.

Scheifele, David W. **37ᵗʰ Annual Meeting of the Infectious Disease Society of America** 1999.

Miller, E, et al., "Idiopathic thrombocytopenic purpura and MMR vaccine", *Archives of Disease of Children* 2001;84:227-229.

Simonsen, L., et al., "Effect of rotavirus vaccination programme on trends in admission of infants to hospital for intussusception", *Lancet* Volume 358, Number 9289 13 October 2001.

Offit, Paul A., M.D., et al.,"Addressing Parents Concerns: Do Multiple Vaccines Overwhelm or Weaken the Infant"s Immune System?", *PEDIATRICS* Vol. 109 No. 1 January 2002, pp. 124-129.

Ball, Leslie K., et al., "An Assessment of Thimerosal Use in Childhood Vaccines", *PEDIATRICS* Vol. 107 No. 5 May 2001, pp. 1147-1154.

Taylor, Brent , et al., "Measles, mumps, and rubella vaccination and bowel problems or developmental regression in children with autism: population study", *BMJ* 2002;324:393-396.

Tucker, Miriam E., "Flu Vaccine Urged For Infants, Families" *Family Practice News* Vol. 32;6:1.

Murphy, Trudy V. M.D., et al., "Intussusception among Infants Given an Oral Rotavirus Vaccine" *New England Journal of Medicine* Volume 344:564-572 February 22, 2001 Number 8.

Daum, Robert S. M.D., et al., "Magnitude of Interference after Diphtheria-Tetanus ToxoidsAcellular Pertussis/*Haemophilus influenzae* Type b Capsular PolysaccharideTetanus Vaccination Is Related to the Number of Doses Administered" *Journal of Infectious Diseases* 2001;184:1293-1299.

Wakefield, A J, M.D., "Ileal-lymphoid-nodular hyperplasia, non-specific colitis, and pervasive developmental disorder in children", *Lancet* 1998; 351: 637-41.

Wakefield, A J, "Autism, inflammatory bowel disease, and MMR vaccine", *Lancet* Volume 351, Number 9106 21 March 1998.

Harald zur Hausen, "Proliferation-inducing viruses in non-permissive systems as possible causes of human cancers", *Lancet* 2001; 357: 381-84.

Vilchez, Regis A, M.D., et. al., "Association between simian virus 40 and non-Hodgkin lymphoma" *Lancet* 2002; 359: 817-23.

Shivapurkar, Narayan, M.D., et al., "Presence of simian virus 40 DNA sequences in human lymphomas" *Lancet* 2002; 359: 851-52.

Lee, et al., 41st Annual Interscience Conference on Antimicrobial Agents and Chemotherapy, "Low varicella vaccine effectiveness identified at day care center", December 2001.

Brisson, M., et al., "Analysis of varicella vaccine breakthrough rates: implications for the effectiveness of immunisation programmes" *Vaccine*, Vol. 18 (25) (2000) pp. 2775-2778.

Chapter II

CONFLICTS OF INTEREST

"Conflicts of Interest and Vaccine Development: Preserving the Integrity of the Process"

Opening Statement
Chairman Dan Burton
Committee on Government Reform
Thursday, June 15, 2000
1:00pm
2154 Rayburn House Office Building
Washington, DC 20515

Today, we are going to continue our series of hearings on vaccine policy. For the last few months, we've been focusing on two important advisory committees. The Food and Drug Administration (FDA) and the Centers for Disease Control and Prevention (CDC) rely on these advisory committees to help them make vaccine policies that affect every child in this country. We've looked very carefully at conflicts of interest. We've taken a good hard look at whether the pharmaceutical industry has too much influence over these committees. From the evidence we found, I think they do.

The first committee is the FDA's Vaccines and Related Biological Products Advisory Committee (VRBPAC). This Committee makes recommendations on whether new vaccines should be licensed. The second committee is the CDC 's Advisory Committee on Immunizations Practices (ACIP). This committee recommends which vaccines should be included on the Childhood Immunization Schedule.

To make these issues easier to understand, we're going to focus on one issue handled by these two committees — the Rotavirus vaccine. It was approved for use by the FDA in August 1998. It was recommended for universal use by the CDC in March 1999. Serious problems cropped up shortly after it was introduced. Children started developing serious bowel obstructions. The vaccine was pulled from the U.S. market in October 1999.

So the question is, was there evidence to indicate that the vaccine was not safe and if so, why was it licensed in the first place? How good a job did the advisory committees do? We've reviewed the minutes of the meetings. At the FDA's committee, there were discussions about adverse events. They were aware of potential problems. Five children out of 10,000 developed bowel obstructions. There were also concerns about children failing to thrive and developing high fevers, which as we know from other vaccine hearings, can lead to brain injury. Even with all of these concerns, the committee voted unanimously to approve it.

At the CDC's committee, there was a lot of discussion about whether the benefits of the vaccine really justified the costs. Even though the cost-benefit ratio was questioned, the Committee voted unanimously to approve it.

Were they vigilant enough? Were they influenced by the pharmaceutical industry? Was there appropriate balance of expertise and perspectives on vaccine issues? We've been reviewing their financial disclosure statements. We've interviewed staff from the FDA and the CDC. The staff has prepared a staff report summarizing what we've found. At the end of my statement, I'll ask unanimous consent to enter this report into the record. We've identified a number of problems that need to be brought to light and discussed.

Families need to have confidence that the vaccines that their children take are safe, effective, and truly necessary. Doctors need to feel confident that when the FDA licenses a drug, that it is really safe, and that the pharmaceutical industry has not influenced the decision-making process. Doctors place trust in the

FDA and assume that if the FDA has licensed a drug, it's safe to use. Has that trust been violated?

How confident in the safety and need for specific vaccines would doctors and parents be if they learned the following:

1. That members, including the Chair, of the FDA and CDC advisory committees who make these decisions own stock in drug companies that make vaccines.

2. That individuals on both advisory committees own patents for vaccines under consideration or affected by the decisions of the committee.

3. That three out of five of the members of the FDA's advisory committee who voted for the rotavirus vaccine had conflicts of interest that were waived.

4. That seven individuals of the 15 member FDA advisory committee were not present at the meeting, two others were excluded from the vote, and the remaining five were joined by five temporary voting members who all voted to license the product.

5.   That the CDC grants conflict-of-interest waivers to every member of their advisory committee a year at a time, and allows full participation in the discussions leading up to a vote by every member, whether they have a financial stake in the decision or not.

6.   That the CDC's advisory committee has no public members — o parents have a vote in whether or not a vaccine belongs on the childhood immunization schedule. The FDA's committee only has one public member.

These are just a few of the problems we found. Specific examples of this include:

Dr. John Modlin—He served for four years on the CDC advisory committee and became the Chair in February 1998. He participated in the FDA's committee as well owned stock in Merck, one of the largest manufacturers of vaccines, valued at $26,000. He also serves on Merck's Immunization Advisory Board. Dr. Modlin was the Chairman of the Rotavirus working group. He voted yes on eight different matters pertaining to the ACIP's rotavirus statement, including recommending for routine use and for inclusion in the Vaccines for Children program. It was not until this past year, that Dr. Modlin decided to divest himself of his vaccine manufacturer stock.

At our April 6 autism hearing, Dr. Paul Offit disclosed that he holds a patent on a rotavirus vaccine and receives grant money from Merck to develop this vaccine. He also disclosed that he is paid by the pharmaceutical industry to travel around the country and teach doctors that vaccines are safe. Dr. Offit is a member of the CDC's advisory committee and voted on three rotavirus issues — including making the recommendation of adding the rotavirus vaccine to the Vaccines for Children's program.

Dr. Patricia Ferrieri, during her tenure as Chair of the FDA's advisory committee, owned stock in Merck valued at $20,000 and was granted a full waiver.

Dr. Neal Halsey, who serves as a liaison member to the CDC committee on behalf of the American Association of Pediatrics, and as a consultant to the FDA's committee, has extensive ties to the pharmaceutical industry, including having solicited and received start up funds from industry for his Vaccine Center. As a liaison member to the CDC committee, Dr. Halsey is there to represent the opinions of the organization he represents, but was found in the transcripts to be offering his personal opinion as well.

Dr. Harry Greenberg, who serves as Chair of the FDA committee, owns $120,000 of stock in Aviron, a vaccine manufacturer. He also is a paid member of the board of advisors of Chiron, another vaccine manufacturer and owns $40,000 of stock. This stock ownership was deemed not to be a conflict and a waiver was granted. To the FDA's credit, he was excluded from the rotavirus discussion because he holds the patent on the rotashield vaccine.

How confident can we be in the process when we learned that most of the work of the CDC advisory committee is done in "working groups" that meet behind closed doors, out of the public eye? Members who can't vote in the full committee because of conflicts of interest are allowed to work on the same issues in working groups, and there is no public scrutiny. I was appalled to learn that at least six of the ten individuals who participated in the working group for the rotavirus vaccine had financial ties to pharmaceutical companies developing rotavirus vaccines.

How confident can we be in the recommendations with the Food and Drug Administration when the chairman and other individuals on their advisory committee own stock in major manufacturers of vaccines?

How confident can we be in a system when the agency seems to feel that the number of experts is so few that everyone has a conflict and thus waivers must be granted. It almost appears that there is a "old boys network" of vaccine advisors that rotate between the CDC and FDA — at times serving simultaneously. Some of these individuals serve for more than four years. We found one instance where an individual served for sixteen years continually on the CDC committee. With over 700,000 physicians in this country, how can one person be so indispensable that they stay on a committee for 11 years?

It is important to determine if the Department of Health and Human Services has become complacent in their implementation of the legal requirements on conflicts of interest and committee management. If the law is too loose, we need to change it. If the agencies aren't doing their job, they need to be held accountable. That's the purpose of this hearing, to try to determine what needs to be done.

Why is this review necessary? Vaccines are the only substances that a government agency mandates a United States citizen receive. State governments have the authority to mandate vaccines be given to children prior to admission to day care centers and schools. State governments rely on the recommendations of the CDC and the FDA to determine the type and schedule of vaccines.

I am not alone in my concern about the increasing influence of industry on medicine. Last year, the *New England Journal of Medicine* learned that 18 individuals who wrote drug therapy review articles had financial ties to the manufacturer of the drugs discussed. The Journal, which has the most stringent conflict of interest disclosures of medical journals, had a recent editorial discussing the increasing level of academic research funded by the industry. The editor stated, "What is at issue is not whether researchers can be 'bought' in the sense of a *quid pro quo,* it is that close and remunerative collaboration with a company naturally creates goodwill on the part of researchers and the hope that the largesse will continue. This attitude can subtly influence scientific judgment."

Can the FDA and the CDC really believe that scientists are more immune to self-interest than other people?

Maintaining the highest level of integrity over the entire spectrum of vaccine development and implementation is essential. The Department of Health and Human Services has a responsibility to the American public to ensure the integrity of this process by working diligently to appoint individuals that are totally without financial ties to the vaccine industry to serve on these and all vaccine-related panels.

No individual who stands to gain financially from the decisions regarding vaccines that may be mandated for use should be participating in the discussion or policy making for vaccines. We have repeatedly heard in our hearings that vaccines are safe and needed to protect the public. If the panels that have made the decisions on all vaccines on the Childhood Immunization Schedule had as many conflicts as we found with rotavirus, then the entire process has been polluted and the public trust has been violated. I intend to find out if the individuals who have made these recommendations that effect every child in this country and around the world, stood to gain financially and professionally from the decisions of the committees they served on.

The hearing record will remain open until June 28 for those who would like to submit a statement into the hearing record.

In a *JAMA*, Editorial, Vol. 284 No. 24, December 27, 2000 "State Mandates and Childhood Immunization" author Kathryn M. Edwards, MD writes...

Routine pediatric immunization programs have eradicated many of the infectious diseases of childhood and have been one of the most remarkable public health accomplishments.

...Why are vaccines under attack? There are several possible explanations. First, cases of vaccine-preventable diseases such as *Bordetella pertussis*, measles, and *Haemophilus influenzae* type b (Hib) meningitis are currently rare, and many parents have never seen or heard of such diseases. Today's parents of young children are too young to have experienced the summer outbreaks of crippling polio, the cases of encephalitis and death during measles epidemics, and the children disabled by Hib meningitis. When faced with more immediate concerns for their children, it is easy for parents to dismiss uncommon infections of years past as being unimportant and their prevention superfluous. Second, with low disease burdens, rates of local and systemic adverse events either causally or temporally related to vaccination appear more common than the diseases themselves. Warnings from the media, on the Internet, and by antivaccine groups that immunizations are dangerous and may lead to autism, seizures, diabetes, or a number of other disorders are disturbing to parents and can contribute to delay or refusal of vaccine administration. That vaccines are required for all children prior to day care or school entry greatly disturbs some parents because they feel that their right to make decisions for their children has been taken away.

Because of these concerns, some state legislators and interest groups are seeking either to repeal state laws mandating vaccination prior to day care or school entry or to provide increased availability of philosophical exemptions for parents who do not want their children immunized. Are legislative mandates necessary to protect children from infectious diseases?

...The findings of Feikin et al are striking. Children aged 3 to 18 years who had exemptions from vaccination were 22 times more likely to acquire measles and nearly 6 times more likely to acquire pertussis than immunized children. In children of day care or primary school age (3-10 years), the risks were more than 60-fold greater for contracting measles and 16-fold greater for pertussis. One might agree that if parents understood these risks, they could choose to accept them for their children and decline immunization. However, the rates of disease among children who were immunized but exposed to children who were exempt from immunization command attention. The annual incidence rates of measles and pertussis among vaccinated children aged 3 to 18 years were significantly associated with frequency of exemptors in that county, with relative risks of 1.6 and 1.9, respectively. The critical issue is whether some parents should be allowed to place other people's children at increased risk for disease by refusing immunizations for their own children.

...In general, the public has been very accepting of immunization laws because it believes that these laws have contributed to disease control in our country. State immunization laws support the priority of vaccines and reinforce their importance. Most parents accept vaccination of their children and realize the health benefits that it affords. To maintain this confidence, it is necessary that states carefully consider each licensed vaccine and use the criteria of severity, contagion, and effectiveness prior to mandating that vaccine for all children. Vaccines remain the most important strategy to prevent infectious diseases in children. We must use our mandates wisely.

Author Affiliation: Department of Pediatrics, Vanderbilt University, Nashville, Tenn.

Corresponding Author and Reprints: Kathryn M. Edwards, MD, Department of Pediatrics, Vanderbilt University Medical Center, D-7221 Medical Center North, Nashville, TN 37232-2581

Financial Disclosure: Dr Edwards has received funding for vaccine studies from Wyeth Lederle, Aventis, SmithKline Beecham, and Merck & Co.

M.E. COMMENTS
Dr. Edwards receives money from drug companies. Is there any way she can be considered an unbiased observer?

Chapter III

CHICKEN POX VACCINE

Chicken Pox Vaccine

Until last year when one of my radio listeners sent
me an article about the manufacturing process, I was
not aware that Varivax, the Chicken Pox Vaccine, is
grown on the cells of aborted fetuses. Merck, one of the
world's largest pharmaceutical companies, very
cleverly uses the words "diploid tissue" instead of
human tissue when they refer to the manufacturing,
production and origin of the Chicken Pox Vaccine.
Diploid is defined by Webster's Medical Dictionary as
"having the basic chromosome number doubled". Only
upon calling Merck did I find out that "diploid tissue"
was human tissue. This human tissue was obtained
from aborted fetuses.

Chicken pox is not necessarily a benign disease.
Complications of chicken pox, in otherwise healthy
children, are rare but they do occur. Chicken pox
complications become even more serious in
adolescents and adults [*The duration of protection of
VARIVAX is unknown, at present, and the need for
booster doses is not defined.*]. Among adults, chicken
pox pneumonia is the most common complication,
resulting in hospitalization in about one in every 400
chicken pox cases. If a vaccine could reduce the
serious complications of chicken pox, ethical and
moral issues aside, this vaccine may be valuable.

However, Merck, in the handout that accompanies
Varivax, states:

> There is insufficient data to assess the rate
> of protection of VARIVAX against the
> serious complications of chicken pox (e.g.,
> encephalitis, hepatitis, pneumonitis) and
> during pregnancy (congenital varicella
> syndrome).
>
> Issued May 1996, Merck & Co. Inc.

In layman's terms what Merck is saying is that
**their Chicken Pox Vaccine, Varivax, does not have
any proven protective effect against the serious
complications of chicken pox.** Since potential
complications could be one of the only medical
justifications for administering the vaccine, based upon
Merck's own statement, there are virtually no medical
indications for the vaccine.

The purpose of a mass inoculation program is not
only to lower the incidence of a disease, but more
importantly to lower the serious side effects or death
rates from that disease. Based on the literature
distributed by Merck, the vaccinated population will
either have the same serious side effects or more
serious side effects. It cannot be assumed from their

literature that the vaccinated population will have less serious side effects.

The following table shows a hypothetical population of 100 people, assuming more side effects in the vaccinated population with a lower incidence of diagnosed chicken pox.

EXAMPLE SHOWING MORE SERIOUS SIDE EFFECTS			
	Diagnosed with Chicken Pox	Serious Side Effects	Death from Side Effects
w/out vaccine	70%	5%	1%
with vaccine	30%	10%	2%

The following table shows a hypothetical population of 100 people, assuming the same number of side effects in the vaccinated population with a lower incidence of diagnosed chicken pox.

EXAMPLE SHOWING EQUAL SIDE EFFECTS			
	Diagnosed with Chicken Pox	Serious Side Effects	Death from Side Effects
with/out vaccine	70%	5%	1%
with vaccine	30%	5%	1%

In our hypothetical population, by using vaccinations the number of diagnosed cases may be lowered; however, the serious side effects and death rate may either be the same or greater. In the vaccinated population, these side effects and death rate may be from the natural disease, or may be a consequence of the vaccine itself.

ೞೞೞೞ

VARIVAX - THE CHICKEN POX VACCINE
Statements made by Merck and Co. about VARIVAX

1) Vaccination may not result in protection of all healthy, susceptible children, adolescents, and adults.

2) The duration of protection of VARIVAX is unknown at present and the need for booster doses is not defined.

3) Each dose of reconstituted vaccine contains trace quantities of neomycin (an antibiotic)

ೞೞೞೞ

Here are a few facts about VARIVAX - most of which can be found right in the manufacturers product insert.

- Individuals vaccinated with Varivax may potentially be capable of transmitting the vaccine virus to close contacts. Therefore, vaccine recipients should avoid close association with susceptible high risk individuals (e.g. newborns, pregnant women, immuno-compromised persons)

- Pregnancy should be avoided for at least 3 months after vaccination

- The long term effect of administering VARIVAX Vaccine on the incidence of herpes zoster (shingles), versus those exposed to natural varicella (chicken pox) is unknown at present

- Physicians advise Varivax vaccine recipients not to use salicylates (aspirin or aspirin containing products) for six weeks after vaccination because of the chance of contracting Reyes syndrome.

- There have been no studies conducted on it for carcinogenic (cancer causing) mutagenic potential or for impairment of fertility.
- This vaccine was cultured in lung tissue obtained from two human aborted fetuses. The vaccine may even contain "residual components "of fetal lung cells.
- No one knows if this will put our children at risk for contracting chicken pox when they become older, when the complications from chicken pox can be more harmful.
- First Year of Vaccine Adverse Events Reporting System (VAERS) based surveillance of the Varicella vaccine has shown over 1,500 reports. Most of the reported categories are rashes, followed by lack of effect, fever, infections, and local injection site reactions. 5% of these reports have been serious including two deaths.

ଔଊଔଊ

Chapter IV

JUST SAY NO TO HEPATITIS B VACCINE

In December 1997, I testified against the proposal by the Illinois Department of Public Health (IDPH) to mandate hepatitis B vaccine for school children. I had already taken the course in Administrative Law in law school so I was familiar with the administration of a governmental agency. The IDPH was under no obligation to be influenced by any of the testimony presented at the hearings. Their only obligation was to hold a hearing. The passage of the mandate for compulsory hepatitis B vaccine for children would be a rubber stamp. This rubber stamping of the hepatitis B mandate did not deter the politically minded and socially conscious, consumer advocate organizations to continue to educate the public with regard to what hepatitis B disease is and to the continuing discovery of more side effects from hepatitis B vaccine.

In October of 1998 the French government ended compulsory hepatitis B vaccine in the French school system. This unique victory came about partially because of an ongoing lawsuit brought by the FNL (French National League for Liberty in Vaccination) against the government of France. Discussing the ruling of the French court in Nanterre, French Health Minister, Bernard Kouchner said "Mass inoculation of school children for hepatitis B has been stopped for fear the vaccine may produce serious neurological disorders." (i.e. Multiple Sclerosis, Chronic Fatigue Syndrome and other degenerative disorders.) In spite of this, health officers from all public health departments (State, Federal and the World Health Organization [WHO]) maintain that the vaccine was safe. The most revealing statement came from the Center for Disease Control (CDC) The CDC stated that hepatitis B vaccine "...is among the safest of vaccines". I found that to be the most revealing statement in all of the discussions and debates. The CDC alleged that the hepatitis B vaccine was among the safest vaccines. If hepatitis B vaccine is among the safest vaccines, which ones are less safe? This admission by the CDC was one of the first acknowledgments that vaccines have risks. It goes against the standard medical establishment party line, "Trust me vaccines are safe and necessary." A poll was conducted by The Chicago Sun-Times after the news release regarding the safety of the hepatitis B vaccine. The question asked was, "Do you want your child vaccinated against hepatitis B?" The results of the poll were shocking. In spite of the insistence by the CDC, WHO, IDPH, and American Academy of Pediatrics (AAP) that the hepatitis B vaccine was safe, 83% of those responding answered the question "NO". Only 17% of those who responded felt they wanted their child vaccinated with hepatitis B vaccine.

I have excerpted some of the preliminary work of Dr. Bonnie Dunbar, Professor of Cell Biology at Baylor College of Medicine (see page 81). Dr. Dunbar has been compiling data on the association between hepatitis B vaccine and Chronic Fatigue Syndrome (CFS), Multiple Sclerosis (MS) and various other auto-immune diseases. Until we get a full disclosure of the risks vs. the benefits it would be foolish to continue a program of mass vaccination. We are the greatest country in the world, partially because we are able to admit our mistakes. I have great faith that as this information about vaccines becomes more widely available, not only will the public reject vaccinations, but the scientists will eventually also reject the unscientific theory of mass immunization programs. I once again call for a moratorium on all childhood vaccinations until we assemble a consensus hearing in Washington, D.C. Let us bring the leading scientists in the related fields together. Let them present the scientific evidence with regard to vaccines. Then let them make a final determination as to the benefits vs. the risk. When presented with the evidence, those NIH Consensus Hearings said NO to fetal monitoring, NO to routine ultrasound, and NO to mammograms for women between ages 40 and 50. Until a final determination is made as to the benefits vs. the risks of vaccines, I as a father, grandfather, and physician will not advocate or administer routine vaccinations. I urge you to say "NO" to the hepatitis B vaccine.

WHO IS AT RISK FOR HEPATITIS B?

[Centers for Disease Control, U.S. Department of Health and Human Services, *Important Information About Hepatitis B Vaccine* 5/27/97. (Distributed by the City of Chicago, Department of Public Health.)]

1) Sexually active adults and teenagers with promiscuous lifestyles.

2) Intravenous drug abusers

3) Children born to mothers who are carriers of hepatitis B

4) Sexually active homosexual men

5) People who get tattoos, ear piercing or body piercing with unsterile needles.

ℭℜℭℜ

Hepatitis B disease should not be confused with hepatitis A disease. These are two separate unique diseases with different modes of transmission.

Hepatitis A can be contracted from contaminated food or contaminated water sources. Hepatitis B disease is only contracted from infected blood sources or sexual relations with people infected with hepatitis B. Hepatitis B is contracted from a risky lifestyle while hepatitis A is a disease which has nothing to do with lifestyle.

Hepatitis B Vaccine developed in 1987, is genetically engineered and is so new that little is known about it. It is not **even** known whether immunity will last until the babies receiving it reach an age when they might engage in high risk sexual activity or drug abuse. Yet, despite the lack of scientific evidence regarding the efficacy of hepatitis B Vaccine, the American Academy of Pediatrics, the Center for Disease Control, and the Illinois Legislature have mandated hepatitis B Vaccine for all children. Hepatitis B Vaccine is routinely given to newborns in virtually all hospitals in this country. Why the "Safe Sex Vaccine" at birth???

CRCRCRCR

Hepatitis B Vaccine - Professor Bonnie Dunbar
Excerpts from Professor Bonnie Dunbar, Professor of Cell Biology, Baylor College of Medicine, as posted on her web page.

Since there is a high probability that hepatitis B vaccine (or the hepatitis B virus itself) may cause MS like symptoms, Dr. Bonnie Dunbar is trying to identify more patients with autoimmune disorders that might be related to the hepatitis B vaccine in order to find a better way to prevent, diagnose, and treat such reactions.

"Within the past two years, I have had two colleagues who have developed severe and apparently permanent adverse reactions as a result of being forced to take the hepatitis B vaccine. Both of these individuals were extremely healthy and very athletic before this vaccine and have had severe, debilitating autoimmune side effects from this vaccine. I know the complete history of one, Dr. Bohn Dunbar, who is my brother who had serious rashes, joint pain, chronic fatigue and now other degenerative disorders including lupus like syndrome and multiple sclerosis like symptoms. One of my medical students went partially blind following her first booster injection and virtually completely blind in one eye following the second hepatitis B vaccine and was hospitalized for several weeks. Following two years of consulting with specialists, the consensus is that Bohn's 'syndromes' are due to adverse reactions to the hepatitis B vaccine.

I have worked in autoimmunity and vaccine development for over twenty years (the past 15 years at Baylor College of Medicine in Houston). I was honored two years ago by the National Institute of Health, as the first Margaret Pittman lecturer, for my pioneering work in contraceptive vaccines. I am, therefore, very sensitive to the balance of risk vs. benefits in vaccine development. Because of my expertise in this area, it became apparent to me that these two active, healthy individuals working in my laboratory at the same time developed "autoimmune" syndromes at the same prolonged immunological time frame following their booster injections of the hepatitis B vaccine. **After carrying out extensive literature research on this vaccine, it is apparent that the serious adverse side effects may be much more significant than generally known.** Because it is not clear that adequate long term follow-up information was collected in the clinical trial data, many of these effects might not have been observed. Even the vaccine insert, which most physicians do not show or discuss with their patients, is ominous.

I have obtained the FDA adverse reaction list of over 8,000 individuals with reported adverse reactions for the past 4 years, this covers the vaccine only. This figure does not include the Smith Kline vaccine, which I have been told includes another 15,000 or more. The vast majority of adults who have these same symptoms including rash, joint pain, chronic fatigue, neurological disorders, neuritis, rheumatoid arthritis, lupus like syndrome and multiple sclerosis like syndrome. (It has been reported by the head of the FDA that these reports indicate only about one tenth of the total numbers of adverse reactions.)

At one point a neurology specialist stated in front of myself and Bohn that 'We are having the same problem with your (Bohn's) diagnosis as we have with vets with Gulf War Syndrome who have the identical symptoms as yours--but there are no definite tests.' In reading various reports on the Gulf War Veterans illnesses, it appears that many of these symptoms are those which are related to the large numbers of adverse reactions reported for the hepatitis B vaccine. It is not clear to me, however, that this vaccine was carefully evaluated as a potential cause of some of these reactions.

French Halt Hepatitis B Vaccine Use

Mon 05 Oct 1998 18:53:00 GMT
PARIS. Oct. 5 (UPI)

French Health Minister Bernard Kouchner says mass inoculation of school children for hepatitis B has been stopped for fear the vaccine may produce serious neurological disorders. Kouchner told French radio this morning some scientific work indicated the possibility that the vaccine might even produce cases of multiple sclerosis, or possibly augment the onset of the affliction. He said, "Problems of the central nervous system and their cause are very complicated and these possibilities must be excluded and that is why we stopped the program."

The mass immunization program began four years ago with inoculation of all 11-year-old children against hepatitis. Earlier this year, a French court in Nanterre ruled there was evidence to show a connection between the vaccine and two people with symptoms of multiple sclerosis.

> ...A statement from WHO officials late
> Friday declared the court decision could
> "lead to loss of public confidence in this
> vaccine, and decisions by other countries

to suspend or delay the introduction of
hepatitis B vaccine." But France has
become especially prudent about such
issues after disclosures its national health
system failed to halt providing
hemophiliacs AIDS-tainted blood products
in the mid-1980s.

M.E. Comments:
*Kudos to the French Government for making the wise
decision eliminating the requirement for hepatitis B
vaccine for school age children. Now, if only our
politicians would be attentive to the findings of the
French government and eliminate mandatory hepatitis
B vaccine as a school requirement. When the Chicago
Sun Times conducted a poll, 83% of the respondents
indicated that they did not want their children
vaccinated with hepatitis B vaccine.*

ღღღღ

Chicago Sun Times
Friday, October 9, 1998

MORNINGLINE
RESULTS
Do you want your child vaccinated against hepatitis B?
YES: 17%   NO: 83%

ෆൣൣ

Adverse Events From Vaccine Said to Outnumber Pediatric Cases of Hepatitis B

WESTPORT, Jan 25, 1999 (Reuters Health) - An advocacy group representing healthcare consumers and the vaccine-injured says that "...the number of hepatitis B vaccine-associated serious adverse event and death reports in American children under 14 outnumber the reported cases of hepatitis B disease in that age group."

The National Vaccine Information Centers calls the government-mandated policy of vaccination of all children against hepatitis B "...dangerous and scientifically unsubstantiated." The US currently mandates a 3-shot series of hepatitis B vaccinations prior to school entry. In October 1998, France ended mandatory vaccination of schoolchildren for hepatitis B because of reports of adverse events.

The organization says that in 1996, there were 872 serious hepatitis B vaccine-associated adverse events reported to the Vaccine Adverse Event Reporting System in children less than 14 years of age. Of these, 214 had received other vaccines at the same time as hepatitis B vaccination.

There were 279 cases of hepatitis B infection in children under the age of 14 in 1996.

CR CR CR CR

Hepatitis B Statistics for All Children in U.S.ALess than 14 Years of Age - 1996	
Cases of hepatitis B Infection	279
Serious hepatitis B vaccine adverse events	872

M.E. Comments:
The reported adverse events from hepatitis B vaccine outnumbered the number of cases of hepatitis B by three to one. It is estimated that only 15% of serious adverse reactions are actually reported. Using this

percentage the actual number of serious adverse events related to hepatitis B vaccine may actually be 5,813.

ଓଃଓଃଓଃଓଃ

FDA Bans Hepatitis B Vaccine Ingredient–
Thimerosal
Actual Letters from the Internet
regarding hepatitis B Vaccine

**Posted by A Mom on the Internet on
January 02, 1999 at 02:52:51:**
Thimerosal (a mercury derived compound) is
an ingredient included in vaccines as a disinfectant and
preservative. Thimerosal is also known to be a
potential cause of brain injury & autoimmune disease.

IN A RULE EFFECTIVE 10-22-98, PUBLISHED IN
FEDERAL REGISTER 63(77):19799-19802, 22 APRIL
1998, THE FDA BANNED USE OF MERCURY AND 15
OF IT'S COMPOUNDS, INCLUDING THIMEROSAL &
MERCUROCHROME, STATING "SAFETY AND
EFFECTIVE-NESS HAVE NOT BEEN ESTABLISHED
FOR THE INGREDIENTS... MANUFACTURERS HAVE
NOT SUBMITTED THE NECESSARY DATA."

The FDA bans Thimerosal from inclusion in over-
the-counter preparations, yet considers direct injection
into our children's bodies as safe and effective? This
type of logic scares me, and it should scare you too!

**Posted on the Internet by Interested on January 04,
1999 at 14:22:30:**

In reply to: <u>FDA bans Hepatitis B Vaccine ingredient</u> posted by A Mom on January 02, 1999 at 02:52:51:

When I was researching the vaccine, My doctor provided me with the drug insert documentation for Engerix-B (the most widely administered [hepatitis B] vaccine). I read it carefully, and if I remember correctly, the ingredient that you reference was listed in its composition as a preservative. So now what ??? Can the drug companies substitute something different, and keep selling the 'stuff', or are they considering halting the program ??? Glad we didn't do this to our kids.

ଔଔଔଔ

Posted by Robin on May 03, 1998 at 12:34:11:

I'm a registered nurse and got multiple sclerosis after my 3rd dose of hep. vac

Looking for healthcare workers noting adverse reactions to the hepatitis B vaccine. Please respond to my email. Thanks

ଔଔଔଔ

Posted by Jayne on December 10, 1998 at 01:41:30:

I went blind with severe optic neuritis within a week of hep B vac. After IV steroids some sight returned but I am still partially sighted. I am a registered nurse. I would like to know if anyone else has had a similar reaction.

ೞೋೞೋ

Posted by Alison on February 27, 1998 at 17:46:03:

I am a health care worker and have had a severe reaction to the Hep, B vaccine I have been researching it for 3 years and you are not alone there are a lot having different types of reactions and the government has added this vaccine to its adverse reaction program. Looking forward to hearing from you. Good health Robin.

෴෴෴

Posted by Peter on June 09, 1998 at 13:48:08:

HFHSM.D-DM on 3 May 1998 in reply to Paula on hep B vaccine side effects who says that because people develop medical problems does not mean that the problem was caused by vaccine. When a medicine or medical procedure is administered, the symptoms experienced must been seen as resulting from the procedure or medicine unless other insult occurred to cause similar symptoms at the time. This is normal medical practice. To try and tell people that their illness was the result of something other then what actually happened is criminal
PB

෴෴෴

Posted by Sheila on June 24, 1998 at 15:44:03:

I am 49 Yrs. Work with mentally handicapped people. In 1989 employer said that all staff needed to be vaccinated for hep. b as we were high risk. I did not know what hepatitis B was. Employer said that the vaccine was completely safe because it was man made, it did not have any of the hepatitis virus in it. The day after the vaccination I was very ill. Could not walk with pains all over body. Employer said that illness was not related to vaccine. Since that time my health has been very bad. Constant infections. Always tired, feel more like 90 then 49. No longer able to play golf, take pictures, enjoy sex. I have recently been diagnosed as having chronic fatigue syndrome. I am in consultation with solicitors and am trying to take legal action against my employer.

CЗСЯСЗСЯ

Posted by Mary Ann on November 22, 1998 at 12:45:48:

Have had severe fatigue, increased sleeping, abdominal discomfort, muscle and joint pain, head-aches and bloating. This is aside from the chronic active hepatitis C I have. I have very severe symptoms i.e. fatigue, muscle, joint and abdominal pain and other. I received the first of the series of the hepatitis A and B vaccines last Tuesday and the above (1st set) of symptoms developed overnight. I can barely move. I hope it wears off.

ᏣᏣᏣᏣ

Chapter V

FLU VACCINE

In 1976, when I just started in my medical practice, one of the great experiments in "modern" medicine took place. The Center for Disease Control predicted a devastating flu epidemic, the "Swine Flu" epidemic. They predicted that thousands of people would die from this strain of flu just as in the flu epidemic of 1918 which caused the deaths of millions of Americans. In order to **"protect"** the American people from this "certain death" the government made the Swine Flu vaccine available free of charge to the public and began administering it at "government vaccine centers". I asked my professor, the late Dr. Robert Mendelsohn, "what should I recommend to my patients, if the government makes this vaccine mandatory?" His response was, "Tell your patients to line up at the back of the line and pray that they run out of vaccine material before your patients reach the front of the line." After just a few weeks, almost 100 people died shortly after being injected with the Swine Flu vaccine and more than 500 people developed Guillain-Barré syndrome (GBS) (see explanation following). The government immediately abandoned the Swine Flu vaccine program. As for the prediction that thousands of people would die from the flu, the total number of cases of Swine Flu was less than 10. This is not the first time that the government and our medical establishment have tried to scare the public into accepting unproven medical treatments. It is no different with hospital birth, bottle feeding, antibiotics, surgery, etc. The argument is always the same, the medical establishment says, "If you do not follow my advice, very bad things will happen to you. Trust me, I am your doctor." The time has come to say, "show me the evidence, show me that the treatment is safer than the disease." Let us get back to the principle espoused by Hippocrates, the father of medicine, "Primum Non Nocere - Above all do no harm," a principle that medicine violates over and over again.

It is my interpretation, according to medical statistics, that the flu vaccine of today is no safer than the Swine Flu vaccine of 1976. The only difference is that in 1976 the flu vaccine was administered to thousands of individuals at government vaccine centers and the data relating to the side effects was readily available. Today, the vaccine is administered in thousands and thousands of doctors offices, work places, drug stores, and grocery stores, with no uniform methodology for reporting accountability or follow up data easily available. Therefore, serious side effects, such as Guillain-Barré Syndrome, are easily missed and the connection is never made. The evidence is not conclusive that the risk of the flu vaccine outweighs the alleged benefits (saving thousands of lives). However, the evidence seems to show that the flu vaccine does have some very serious side effects.

At this time, we need to call for a moratorium on all vaccinations. We need to convene a panel of the leading experts in medicine. This panel must be devoid of sponsorship from any drug companies or parties that have any vested interest in the outcome. The panel should review all the scientific articles and data on vaccinations. Afterwards, they should make their recommendations. It is very interesting that whenever the National Institute of Health has convened such consensus panels the results are far different than we would expect. In the past, these NIH consensus panels have recommended fewer ultra sounds, fewer breast cancer surgeries, less cesarean sections, and they have questioned routine mammograms for women. I have great faith in the honesty of scholarly physicians. When they meet in large consensus groups and review data they come to unbiased conclusions relying on the information presented to them and not relying on political agendas, or their own beliefs.

At the present time, your doctor will try to scare you about the flu, until all the evidence is in, Mayer

Eisenstein, M.D., will scare you about the flu vaccine. My advice is say "No" to the flu vaccine. If you get the flu ask your grandmother for her chicken soup recipe!

The following information was learned over the many years that I was a student of Dr. Mendelsohn. See page xii.

> "The mad vehemence of Modern Medicine is nowhere more evident than in the yearly influenza vaccine farce. I can never think about flu shots without remembering a wedding I once attended. Strangely enough, no grandparents were among the participants and no one seemed to be over age 60. When I finally asked where all the old folks were, I was told they had all received their flu shots a few days before. They were all at home recovering from the shots' ill effects!

> The entire flu shot effort resembles some massive roulette game, since from one year to the next it's anybody's guess whether the strains immunized against will be the strains that are epidemic. We were all afforded a peek at the real

dangers of flu vaccines when in 1976, the Great Swine Flu Fiasco revealed, under close government and media surveillance, 565 cases of Guillain-Barré paralysis resulting from the vaccine and thirty "unexplained" deaths of older persons within hours after receiving the shot. I wonder what would be the harvest of disaster if we kept as close a watch on the effects of all the other flu shot campaigns. Dr. John Seal, of the National Institute of Allergy and Infectious Disease says, "We have to go on the basis that any and all flu vaccines are capable of causing Guillain-Barré syndrome."

ଓଃଓଃ

ONE FLU OVER THE CUCKOO'S NEST
http://www.4icpa.org/research/vaccinat.htm
"Vaccine enthusiasts reached the height of their folly in 1976 when a pandemic of "killer Swine Flu" was predicted. America was asked to buy a "pig in a poke" and accept vaccination. The media proclaimed that failure to do so would result in an epidemic that would rival any in recorded

history. The government spent millions on the vaccine. The outcome: There were deaths. There were cases of paralysis, but they were not from the dreaded "killer flu." They resulted from the vaccine that was supposed to prevent it.

J. Anthony Morris, one time head of influenza control in the U.S. warned his superiors in the federal government that the vaccine was dangerous and probably ineffective. When they refused to act, he went directly to the media. Morris advised the public that the vaccine was unsafe, and an epidemic was unlikely. As a result, he was fired from his position at the Food and Drug Administration. His experimental animals, representing years of research, were destroyed. Publication of his findings was blocked by his superiors.

Other scientists and physicians were also critical of the vaccine. Nobel Laureate, Linus Pauling, in a letter to the first author dated May 11, 1976, indicated that he and his wife did not intend to take the vaccine because he felt there was "significant dangers" associated with it. The Lancaster, Pennsylvania *Intelligencer Journal* of August 14, 1976 reported on a survey of practicing physicians asked about the vaccine. 100 percent of the physicians surveyed said they would not administer Swine Flu shots to their own children. T.A. Vonder Haar, then Coordinator of Programs in Public Policy at the University of Missouri, stated in a letter dated May 10, 1976. "Virus vaccines are notoriously ineffective...flu vaccines have been documented as having contained SV.40, a known carcinogen, with full FDA knowledge."

Even the insurance industry balked at this one. They refused to indemnify vaccine makers against claims arising from the administration of Swine Flu vaccine. C. Joseph Stetler, then president of the Pharmaceutical Manufacturer's Association was quoted by UPI as saying, "It's like you taking out a life insurance policy and suddenly becoming a kamikaze pilot." The answer — the government

agreed to insure the vaccine makers! What
was the result of this debacle?

According to Newsweek, July 18, 1977,
$135 million was appropriated by
Congress to indemnify vaccine makers.
However, claims totaling over $1.3 billion
dollars were filed with the Justice
Department alleging injury or death as a
result of the Swine Flu shots. 517
Americans were stricken with Guillain-
Barré syndrome, and at least 23 died. And
what of the killer epidemic? The total
number of Swine Flu cases was six, and in
some cases the diagnosis was
questionable.

Are things better today? A common ritual
in America is getting a flu shot "just in
case" when "flu season" is imminent. How
safe and effective are today's influenza
vaccines? Scheifle et. al. in a study
reported in the *Canadian Medical
Association Journal,* January 15, 1990,
described the results of hospital workers
receiving trivalent influenza vaccine
prepared for the 1988-1989 flu season...

"Of approximately 500 full-time workers in 'high risk' areas, 288 took the vaccine. Of these, 266 returned a questionnaire regarding any symptoms experienced within 48 hours after the vaccination. 90 percent of the respondents reported adverse effects. 49 percent reported systemic adverse effects. Five percent missed work as a consequence of vaccine adverse effects."

ෆිෆිෆිෆි

Guillain-Barré Syndrome

Guillain-Barré (*ghee yan-bah ray*) **Syndrome**, (**GBS**) is a rare and unpredictable syndrome which causes the person's life to go into utter chaos and turmoil. This syndrome, is also called *acute idiopathic polyneuritis*, a disorder that consists of weakness and even paralysis of many of the body's muscles, along with abnormal sensations. The illness can be present in several ways, at times making the diagnosis difficult to establish in its early stages. The specific cause is not known. Research to date indicates that, the nerves of the person who has Guillain-Barré, are attacked by the body's defense system against disease (antibodies and white blood cells). As a result of this attack, the nerve insulation (myelin) and sometimes even the covered conducting part of the nerve (axon) is damaged. This causes delay or change of the nerve "messages", between the sender (usually the brain, cortex or spinal column) and receiver (usually a muscle). The abnormal sensations and weakness quickly follow.

CSCRCSCR

Judge loses use of hands, legs
Chicago Sun Times - Wed., February 4, 1998

"The chief judge of Will County Circuit Court has been diagnosed with Guillain-Barré syndrome, an illness that has left him unable to use his hands and legs.

Herman Hasse, 55, became ill two weeks ago while attending a judicial conference in Miami.

Hasse had flu-like symptoms before leaving and family members told him the illness might have been triggered by a flu shot. The Illinois Department of Health said there is no statistically significant risk of getting the syndrome from a flu shot."

⊗⊗⊗⊗

GBS and Flu Shot
Responses posted on the Internet:
Submitted by Teresa on 6/30/98.

Would like to know about death from GBS, 2 wk incubation period from flu shot, symptoms, etc. my dad just died mysteriously, had many symptoms of GBS, but had recently had a flu shot. His immune system was very poor, overall physical and mental health was poor.

Submitted by Doris on 2/22/98.
My husband and I were told 2 things:

> 1 - The neurologist and immunologist who treated Steve told him that they would personally never get another vaccine if they were him UNLESS it was life threatening.

> 2 - At a MD Chapter meeting in Nov '97, Dr Carol Koski, head of Neurology at Univ of MD, was asked about the flu shot and GBS. She said GBS patients should refrain from getting the flu shot for one year after getting GBS. After that, she saw no reason why the annual flu shot couldn't be resumed.

> On a personal basis, my husband Steve came down with GBS in '96 - in Oct '95 he rec'd his first flu shot. In Jan '96 he rec'd a cocktail of shots for an overseas trip. Could there be a connection ?

CR&CR&CR&CR&

Submitted by Steve on 5/24/98.
I got GBS in 1981 shortly after taking the flu shot. I never took the shot again for years. I finally decided to take the flu shot

again in the mid-90's. I think I took it two or three times with no GBS. But, in '96, I took the shot and soon thereafter developed a bad rash on my abdomen. A short time later, I developed GBS again. I am not sure if the rash was connected, but I am personally convinced that the flu shot and GBS are connected in my case. I will never take the shot again, and my neurologist agreed.

ଓଔଓଔ

A Personal Story Guillain Barré After Flu Vaccine as posted on the Internet.

Ray's story...

Wife Martha & I had experienced flu attacks in January 1994 & 1995. Nothing severe - just put us to bed except to get up for something to eat once each day for about a week. Low-grade fever, aching, continuing cough, etc. However, there are more pleasant things so we decided in the fall of '95 to undergo the flu shot - neither of us had had one for at least 40 years. I was 63 and retired. Have had blood pressure problems for 25 years & some heart arrhythmia, but no general symptoms and pretty much do as I wish (had never been hospitalized a day in my life).. We both received one injection of Parke-Davis' "Fluogen" vaccine. Were told to come for a second one in two weeks since it had been so long since being vaccinated. Neither of us have returned for that second shot, nor will we ever do so.

I assume we were given vaccine from the same vial. I went first and noticed the nurse agitating the vial. I could see thru the liquid against the backlight of the fridge interior light and noticed some light particulate moving thru the liquid. I know some vaccines appear this way & was not concerned. Martha was injected in the upper left arm and had some soreness for several days. My injection was to the upper left muscle on top of the shoulder. The only effect I noted was the other shoulder muscle was a little sore the next day. The shots were given on 9/21/95. Martha had no further problems. On 10/1/95 I awoke with everything tasting as if I had a mouthful of salt. This went on all day. On the morning of 10/2/95 I noticed that everything tasted bad (no longer salty). Even water tasted strange. Later I went to the bathroom to wash my hands and started in cold water - it felt hot. When it warmed to lukewarm it was excruciating. Carpal tunnel syndrome had returned to my wrists. This had not bothered during the seven years since my retirement. Later that afternoon I went to check the mailbox feeling okay, but was so weak on the return trip I barely made it back into the house. Never mind - all will be well tomorrow.

On the morning of 10/3/95 Martha had to pull me out of bed. I could not get to a sitting position even by extending my legs over the side of the bed and using them as a counter-weight. Went to the bathroom to prepare for a doctor visit and somehow wound up on the floor unable to get up. With my arms extended backward behind me and bouncing on my backside I managed to get to the den. By placing my hands on the low couch behind me and pushing hard with my feet & legs was able to get to a setting position on the couch. As

I dressed Martha pulled the car across the sidewalk just beyond the porch & left the door open. With my hands on her shoulders, I was able to rise from the couch and follow her to the car.

Having called in advance the doctor's office met me with a wheelchair. Wheeled into an examining room, first check was blood pressure - over the moon. Had tried to check it the night before but could not get my machine pumped high enough to get a systolic (upper) reading & assumed the machine was broken. They immediately arranged a hospital room (just across the driveway) & I was wheeled over & checked in.

Two days of testing which included blood work-ups, urinalyses, X-rays, CAT scan & MRI I was finally diagnosed with a spinal tap which revealed high protein in the spinal fluid. Evaluation was AIDP & it was on to ICU. About the third day in ICU my breathing declined & I was ventilated. In the 30 days in ICU (15 with the ventilator in place) I would estimate my conscious time at not more than 2 hours and that was marginal. I was pronounced paraplegic at one point, being able to move only my toes very slightly. Plasmapheresis (plasma exchange) did nothing for me. However, three small infusions of IVIG (intravenous immunoglobulin) & body movement returned. A fourth infusion did very little and the fifth was canceled. I came to in Rehab a day later with some slight paralysis to both hands but was told I would be unable to walk. In my first trip to Physical Therapy I could not even rise to stand on the parallel bars (too weak from 30 days with no food other than albumin 5% on the IV. However, on the second day I rose & walked the length of the bars. Two days later I was on the walker and I walked from the hospital without aid on the 21st day of Rehab. I am left with feet which still feel stiff (they are not), good walking ability on smooth surfaces (not so good on rough or slanted terrain), hands that are sometimes a little stiff and tingle, as do the feet. In ICU I encountered blood pressures in the high

200's and as low as 34 (deadly). I encountered 5 blood clots which had to be dissolved and had a vena cava filter installed to catch any clot fragments which entered the bloodstream. This will remain for the balance of my life.

Guillain-Barré Syndrome is a dangerous, potentially deadly condition with long-term after effects. Persons contemplating the influenza shot should be made aware that this is an always present possibility, and need to realize that GBS is not some mild reaction, but is rather a hard paralysis capable of bringing on disability, severe illness and death.

ଔଔଔଔ
"Revaccinations Not Necessary After Flu Vaccine Recall"

OLYMPIA, Wash.--February 13, 1997-- Parke-Davis today recalled all remaining lots of its Fluogen influenza due to a decrease in potency.

The vaccine was recalled after tests conducted by Parke-Davis showed that the potency of the vaccine was decreasing, and may not adequately protect recipients against the strains of influenza that had been seen this season.

M.E. Comments:

The ineffectiveness of the Fluogen influenza vaccine to protect against influenza, did not prevent Ray from developing GBS.

ଓଔଓଔ

The Flu Vaccine Is It Really Safe and Effective? What Is In A Flu Vaccine?

Formaldehyde: a known cancer causing agent Thimerosal: (a mercury derivative) used as a preservative in the vaccine, can cause brain injury and autoimmune disease.   Also this vaccine is propagated on chicken embryo cells.

The problem with using animal cells is that during serial passage of the virus thru the animal cells, animal RNA and DNA can be transferred from one host to another. Undetected animal viruses may slip past quality control testing procedures (see page xv).

In 1995 a team of Swiss scientists discovered an enzyme, reverse transcriptase. Keep in mind reverse transcriptase copies RNA and DNA and is associated with retroviruses in MMR vaccines and some influenza vaccines that had been propagated in chicken embryo .

ଓଃଠଃଠଃଠ

How Effective is the Vaccine?

Flu vaccine production is a big guessing game. Every year the CDC has to try and predict what virus will infect people in the U.S. the following year. This is something like looking thru a crystal ball. So how accurate is this crystal ball?

In 1992-93 the isolated influenza samples for the predominant virus (influenza A (H3N2) virus) were not similar to that in the vaccine (MMWR 42 752-55).

In the 1994-95 influenza season the CDC reported that 43% of isolated influenza samples for the predominant virus were not similar to the vaccine. The same goes for another type A virus (HINI) and the influenza B they also were not similar to that in the vaccine (MMWR 9/8/95).

In a 1993 Dutch article on a nursing home for the elderly, 50% of the vaccinated population contracted the illness compared to 48% of the unvaccinated.

Vaccine efficiency in elderly is usually never higher then 52-67%. Other doctors and studies declare it even lower, showing an efficiency rate of 20% or less and if you keep in mind mistakes in production, transport, and storage this may even cause a further decrease in effectiveness.

ദ്രദ്രദ്രദ്ര

How Safe are Flu Vaccines?

We have all heard of the Swine Flu Vaccine disaster of 1976 that caused over 565 cases of Guillain-Barré Syndrome paralysis, as well as other neurological problems and many unexplained deaths among recently vaccinated elderly.

Although vaccine manufacturers try to say today's vaccines do not carry the same risk of Guillain Barré Syndrome as was caused by the Swine Flu vaccine, many cases (as well as other neurological problems) are still occurring after flu vaccines. In the early 1980's Dr. John Seal of the National Institute of Allergy and Infectious Disease stated that "We have to go on the basis that any and all flu vaccines are capable of causing Guillain-Barré."

Flu vaccine product inserts do state that individuals who have a history of Guillain-Barré Syndrome have a substantially greater likelihood of subsequently developing GBS.

In 1970, G.A. Rosenberg, in an article in the New England Journal of Medicine, wrote about meningoencephalitis being reported as a result of influenza vaccines. He then goes on to describe a case of a patient in which meningoencephalitis developed 12 days after vaccination with a purified influenza vaccine.

Other reactions that have been associated with past influenza vaccines are: fever,

malaise, myalgia, hives, angioedema,
allergic asthma, systemic anaphylaxis,
Guillain- Barré Syndrome, encephalo-
pathy, optic neuritis, brachial plexus
neuropathy, many different types of
paralysis, myletitis polyneuritis (including
cases of polyradiculitis, polyradiculo-
myelitis, and polyganglioradiculitis),
ataxia, respiratory infections,
gastro-intestinal problems, eye problems,
allergic thrombocytopenia, disturbed
blood pressure, collapse, etc.

ଔଓଔଓ

REFERENCES - Chapters III-V

Center For Complex Infectious Diseases -
  http://www.ccid.org/
  John Martin, M.D., Ph.D. - Web Site
  This site provides information on stealth viruses.
  The issue of live viral vaccines as a probable
  source of certain stealth viruses and a known
  source of SV40 virus is also addressed.

Centers for Disease Control and Prevention -
  http://www.cdc.gov/ncidod/diseases/flu/fluvac.ht
  m

Concerned Parents for Vaccine Safety's Home Page -
  http://home.sprynet.com:80/sprynet/Gyrene/

Department of Neurology at Massachusetts General
  Hospital http://neuro-www.mgh.harvard.
  edu/forum/GuillainBarreSyndromeMenu.html

GBS Syndrome -
  http://terri.adsnet.com/jsteinhi/html/gbs/gbsmain
.html

Hepatitis B Vaccine Study -
  http://webpages.netlink.co.nz/~ias/dunbar.htm
  Dr. Bonnie S. Dunbar, PhD, Professor,
  Department of Cell Biology Baylor College of
  Medicine, has identified patients with
  autoimmune disorders that might be related to
  the hepatitis B vaccine in order to find a better
  way to prevent, diagnose, and treat such

reactions. Since it is clearly established that this vaccine (or the virus infection itself) may cause multiple sclerosis like symptoms, further information could be a great help for her ongoing research.

How Safe Is Universal Hepatitis B Vaccination? - **www.waisbrenclinic.com**
Burton A. Waisbren, Sr., M.D., F.A.C.P. - Web Site
In this scholarly paper Dr. Waisbren discusses four of the theories with regard to the association between hepatitis B vaccine and adverse neurological findings (i.e. multiple sclerosis, chronic fatigue syndrome, Guillain-Barré, etc.)

ILLINOIS VACCINE AWARENESS COALITION (IVAC)
http://www.vaccineawareness.org/
P.O. Box 946, Oak Park, IL 60303
Phone: (708) 848-0116
Barbara Alexander Mularkey
Call or write for outstanding information on vaccines.

Mendelsohn, Robert S. M.D., How To Raise A Healthy Child... In Spite of Your Doctor, Contemporary Books, Inc., Chicago.

Mendelsohn, Robert S. M.D., Confessions of a Medical Heretic, 1979, Contemporary Books.

National Vaccine Information Center (NVIC) -
  http://www.909shot.com/
  An outstanding site for information on
  vaccinations. A must!

Ohio Parents for Vaccine Safety
  251 West Ridgeway Drive, Dayton, OH 45459
  Phone: (937) 435-4750
  Christine M. Severyn, R.Ph., Ph.D., Director
  Call or write for outstanding newsletters on
  vaccines, as well as complimentary information.

Vaccine Information & Awareness -
  http://www.access1.net/via/
  VIA empowers parents to question, challenge,
  investigate, research, and become more informed
  and aware about the risks and dangers that exist
  with vaccines.

Tetrahedron -
  www.tetrahedron.org
  Dr. Len Horowitz - Web Site
  This web site will be of interest to all those who
  want to be better informed of the risks of
  childhood vaccines. Dr. Horowitz points the
  finger at contaminated vaccines as a potential
  cause of AIDS, Ebola, Asthma, Chronic fatigue,
  Depression, Colitis, Diabetes, Breast Cancer,
  Prostate Cancer, and others.

Vaccination? The Choice is Yours! -
  http://www.avn.org.au/

"In light of the high public regard for medicine, it may come as a surprise that modern medical techniques such as vaccinations and antibiotics have had no significant impact on the overall death rate in industrialized societies during the past century. Death rates in these societies have certainly declined sharply - but they did so before the introduction of vaccinations and antibiotics."

www.homefirst.com - go to vaccine links.

Chapter VI

CONFIDENTIALITY
TRADITIONAL MEDICAL/MODERN
MEDICAL VS.
LEGAL PROFESSIONAL
RESPONSIBILITIES

Confidentiality

<u>The Hypothetical Case</u>
　　　A parent brings a six month old child to a physician for an upper respiratory infection. The physician questions the parent about the child's vaccine history. The parent, assuming that this communication is privileged and confidential, replies that they have not made a final decision about administering the childhood vaccines. At the present time their child has not received any of the childhood vaccines.

　　　What is the medical/ethical responsibility of the physician with this in regard to the medical confidential disclosure about childhood vaccines? How would this be treated using traditional medical ethics vs. modern medical ethics vs. legal ethics? The traditional medical oaths (Hippocratic Oath[1] & Oath of Geneva[2]) did not allow the physician to reveal a confidential communication from his patient. Today, the AMA (American Medical Association) "Allows confidential statements to be revealed in instances

---

　　　[1] Internet - http://www.forthnet.gr/asclepeion/hippo.htm

　　　[2] *World Medical Journal 3* (1956), Supplement, pp. 10-12.

when the law allegedly allows it, even if it is not in the best medical interests of the patient."[3] The "Code of Professional Legal Responsibility" only allows the revealing of confidential information if the lawyer believes or suspects that there is a potential for imminent death or substantial bodily harm without the revealing of this confidential communication.[4]

The Law

The Illinois law states that all children must be vaccinated unless they have a medical or religious exemption.[5] Does non-compliance with the law constitute child neglect as described in 325 ILCS 5/3?

Definitions
325 ILCS 5/3 - "Neglected Child"

> "Neglected child" means any child who is not receiving the proper or necessary nourishment or medically indicated

---

[3] *The Illinois Practice of* Family Law 1996-97 Edition, Davis, Muller, West Publishing Company, St. Paul, MN 1996.

[4] *1997 Selected Standards on Professional Responsibility*, Morgan & Rotunda, The Foundation Press, Inc., Westbury, NY 1997.

[5] 410 ILCS 315/2.

treatment... as determined by a physician acting along or in consultation with other physicians or otherwise is not receiving the proper or necessary support or medical or other remedial care recognized under State law as necessary for a child's well being.

325 ILCS 5/4 - "Persons Required to Report; Medical personnel; Privileged communications...

Any Physician... having reasonable cause to believe a child known to them in their professional or official capacity may be an abused child or a neglected child shall immediately report or cause a report to be made to the department... the privileged quality of communication between any professional person required to report and his patient or client shall not apply to situations involving abused or neglected children and shall not constitute grounds for failure to report as required by this Act.

"Required reporting. Medical and mental health professionals and others covered by the Act (the Act does not include lawyers),

are required to immediately make a report
to the Illinois Department of Child and
Family Services. The physician-patient
privilege does not excuse a professional
required to report under the Act from
reporting knowledge of incidents of child
abuse or neglect." [6]

In order to compare medical vs. legal/professional
responsibility, we will compare traditional vs. modern
medical oaths, against the standard of legal
professional responsibility.

<u>The Medical Oaths</u>
The following is a comparison of the Hippocratic
Oath, Oath of Geneva, and the American Medical
Association Principles of Medical Ethics and the
Standard of Legal Professional Responsibility.

<u>The Hippocratic Oath</u>
The Hippocratic Oath embodies one of the oldest
codes of medical ethics. The principles which it
supports have only slightly changed regardless of place,
time, social systems or religious beliefs. The Oath,

---

[6] *The Illinois Practice of* Family Law 1996-97
Edition, Davis, Muller, West Publishing Company, St.
Paul, MN 1996.

written in the 5th Century B.C., has until recently been taken by graduates of medical schools all over the world.

> I SWEAR by Apollo the physician and Aesculapius, and Health, and All-heal, and all the gods and goddesses, that, according to my ability and judgment... Whatever in the connection with my professional service, or not in connection with it, I see or hear, in the life of men, which ought not to be spoken of abroad... **I will not divulge, as reckoning that all such should be kept secret.**[1]

Oath of Geneva

Adopted by the General Assembly of the World Medical Association at Geneva in 1948 and amended by the 22nd World Medical Assembly at Sydney in 1968, the Declaration Of Geneva was one of the first and most important actions of the Association. It is a declaration of physicians' dedication to the humanitarian goals of medicine, a declaration that was especially important in view of the medical crimes

---

[1] Internet - http://www.forthnet.gr/asclepeion/hippo.htm

which had just been committed in Nazi Germany. The Declaration of Geneva was intended to update the Oath of Hippocrates, which the Assembly thought was no longer suited to modern conditions.

> At the time of being admitted as a member of the medical profession:

> I solemnly pledge myself to consecrate my life to the service of humanity;... The health of my patient will be my first consideration;... **I will respect the secrets which are confided in me**, even after the patient has died;... I will not use my medical knowledge contrary to the laws of humanity.[2]

American Medical Association Principles of Medical Ethics

> **Preamble:** The medical profession has long subscribed to a body of ethical statements developed primarily for the benefit of the patient. As a member of this profession, a physician must recognize responsibility not only to patients, but also

---

[2] *World Medical Journal 3* (1956), Supplement, pp. 10-12.

to society, to other health professionals, and to self. The following principles adopted by the American Medical Association are not laws, but standards of conduct which define the essentials of honorable behavior for the physician.

...III. A physician shall respect the law and also recognize a responsibility to seek changes in those requirements which are contrary to the best interests of the patient.

IV. A physician shall respect the rights of patients, of colleagues, and of other health professionals, and shall **safeguard patient confidences within the constraints of the law.**[3]

As opposed to the Hippocratic Oath and the Oath of Geneva, the American Medical Association has abandoned the concept of absolute privilege to the confidential statements made between doctor and

---

[3] *American Medical Association* Council on *Ethical and Judicial Affairs Code of Medical Ethics: Current Opinions and Annotations.* 1996-1997 Edition.

patient. The AMA allows confidential statements to be revealed, in instances when the law allegedly allows it, even if it is not in the best interest of the patient, thus breaking the sacred bond of "confidentiality".

<u>Legal Professional Responsibility</u>
RULE 1.6 Confidentiality of Information

    (a) A lawyer shall not reveal information relating to representation of a client unless the client consents after consultation, except for disclosures that are impliedly authorized in order to carry out the representation, and except as stated in paragraph (b).

    (b) A lawyer may reveal such information to the extent the lawyer reasonably believes necessary:

        (1) to prevent the client from committing a criminal act that the lawyer believes is likely to result in imminent death or substantial bodily harm;[7]

---

[7] *1997 Selected Standards on Professional Responsibility,* Morgan & Rotunda, The Foundation

We see that the Code of Professional Legal Responsibility only allows the revealing of confidential information between lawyer/client where there is threat of imminent death or substantial bodily harm.

When we were in grammar school the revealing of secrets to third parties was called snitching or tattletalling. This behavior carried with it the highest level of disgust. The greatest respect was given to fellow classmates who even in the face of punishment would not reveal a "privileged communication". The drastic change in the field of medical ethics with regard to revealing confidential communications has led to the following satirical contemporary version of the Hippocratic Oath

The Corporate Physician's Oath

I swear by Humana and Columbia HCA and Cigna and Prudential and FHP and Wellpoint and HMO and PPO and IPA making them my witnesses, that I will fulfill according to my ability this oath and this covenant:

Press, Inc., Westbury, NY 1997.

...Things which I may see or hear in the course of treatment, or even outside of treatment regarding the life of human beings, things which one should never divulge outside, I will report to government commissions, immigration officials, hospital administrators, or use in my book.

If I fulfill this oath and do not violate it, may it be granted to me to enjoy life and business, being able to retire at age 50 in the sunbelt. If I transgress it and swear falsely, may Milwaukee be my lot. [8]

The once noble profession of medicine has now succumbed, in its moral and ethical dealings, to corporate medicine. No longer is the patient's health a doctor's first consideration.

---

[8] *New England Journal of Medicine*, January 2, 1986, revised by David Schiedermayer, May 27, 1995.

Confidentiality

We return to the physician in the emergency room seeing the patient with the upper respiratory infection. The doctor is faced with an ethical dilemma. How shall he interpret the Illinois law with regard to childhood vaccinations? If the physician feels that not vaccinating a child constitutes child medical neglect, he is obligated by Illinois law to report these parents to the Department of Child and Family Services (DCFS). However, even if the physician feels that not vaccinating a child constitutes child medical neglect, he has an ethical obligation as stated in the Oath of Hippocrates, as well as in the Oath of Geneva, to maintain absolute secrecy about this privileged communication. The family has not made a final decision about childhood vaccinations. Also, at the present time, the action of the parents not to vaccinate at this time is not likely to result in imminent death or substantial bodily harm. (*The legal standard for revealing confidential communications.*) That leaves the physician with his own ideological thinking about revealing confidential communications. If the physician follows the Hippocratic Oath or the Oath of Geneva, irrespective of his feelings with regard to childhood vaccines, he will keep this communication secret and privileged. However, if the physician follows the AMA Standard of Ethics, he will feel obligated to report the parents to the

DCFS and the parents may lose custody of their child over the issue of childhood vaccines.

The legal profession has maintained a very high standard with regard to protecting privileged lawyer/client communications. This allows the client to reveal virtually everything to his lawyer without worrying about the consequences of the communication. This is in contrast to the erosion of the physician/patient confidentiality, which has led to patients not being able to communicate fully with their physician and thereby not allowing the physician to administer the best possible medical care.

What you Say *Can* Be used Against You
Many consumers believe their medical records are protected, and they'd be surprised to learn just how many organizations have access to their files. Under existing laws, our financial records and even lists of videos we rent have more protection than our health records. In the medical arena, security is spotty, especially after files leave a doctor's office to be examined by insurers, researchers, auditors and drug marketers.

This dearth of protection is having a chilling effect on the doctor-patient relationship. Afraid that insurers or employers will use medical information against them, cautious consumers are becoming wary of disclosing to doctors necessary information about patterns of tobacco and alcohol use, risky sexual behavior, domestic abuse or even a family history of disease.

They Know Who You Are - Jean Fourcroy, M.D., (a urologist in Bethesda MD, and former president of the American Medical Women's Association) and others report that the privacy problem may soon get worse. The Health Insurance Portability and Accountability Act of 1996 (formerly known as the Kennedy-Kassenbaum bill) calls for the creation of a national system of universal patient identifiers: an ID number, similar to a social security number, that will allow all of an individual's health records to be called up on a computer by anyone who treats her.[9]

As physicians, we must look to the legal code of professional responsibility and once again go back to the days when doctor/patient communication was as sacred as communication between lawyer/client, i.e. absolute secrecy unless it is likely to result in imminent death or substantial bodily harm. Otherwise, as physicians, we will be no better than the physicians in Nazi Germany whose excuse for their behavior was "we were just following orders". With a return to the principle of absolute privilege and confidential communication we may be able to repair the eroded confidence that patients have in their physicians.

---

[9] *American Health for Women* magazine, Sandroff, Ronni, July/August 1997.

Chapter VII

VACCINE LAW

At the present time, all 50 states in the United States allow for medical exemption to childhood vaccines. With the exception of West Virginia and Mississippi all states also allow for a religious exemption to childhood vaccines. Currently 17 states have philosophical exemptions to vaccines. Since vaccine mandates are state determined, vaccine laws may vary from state to state. Before submitting any medical, philosophical or religious exemption documentation, I recommend reviewing your state law with an attorney to see which is applicable in your state.

Illinois Medical Exemption From Mandated Childhood Vaccine

Illinois law allows for medical, as well as religious, exemptions from childhood vaccinations, but not a philosophical exemption. Section 665.520 of the Illinois Administrative Code states:

a)   Any medical objection to an immunization must be

1) Made by a physician licensed to practice medicine in all its branches indicating what the medical condition is.

          2) Endorsed and signed by physician on
the certificate of child health examination
and placed on file in the child's permanent
record.

b)   Should the condition of the child later
permit immunization, this requirement
will then have to be met.

The Illinois Administrative Law has given the Illinois
Department of Public Health the right to question your
physician's medical assessment and substitute its own
physician. With an abundance of scientific studies
pointing to the safety of vaccines, even though there are
as many studies pointing out the adverse effects, it is
unlikely that the physician they appoint to consult with
will find medical contraindications to any of the
mandated childhood vaccines.

Illinois Religious Exemption to Vaccines

A search of the medical literature shows that there are
as many scientific studies pro vaccine as anti-vaccine.
Therefore, to argue that vaccines should or should not
be given based on scientific medical grounds, is not
definitive.

Section 665.510 of the Illinois Administrative Code states that:

> "The religious objection must set forth the specific religious belief which conflicts with the examination, immunization or other medical intervention."

The specific religious objection may be personal or it may be directed by the tenets of an established religious organization. The Illinois case law has held that the objection does not have to be written on church stationary, nor does it have to be signed by a rabbi, priest or minister, physician or attorney, etc. In statutory interpretation there are key words that comprise the elements of the statute. With regard to religious exemption under Illinois vaccine law the key words are **specific, personal** and **tenets**.

You must *specifically* state your sincere religious belief. The word specific in the law is open to interpretation. It most probably means that religious or biblical references have brought you to that conclusion. It does not mean that you believe that vaccines are medically dangerous and therefore God does not intend for you to give them. That argument would be construed a medical exemption - not as a religious exemption. A religious exemption implies that even if the vaccines are shown to be 100% safe and are effective you would still object on religious grounds.

Your belief must be directed by the *tenets* of an established religious organization.

If you belong to a recognized religious organization whose tenets speak against childhood vaccinations, you should present a document stating that you are a member of that religious organization.

***Or* it may be your *personal* religious belief.**

The religious beliefs may be personal religious beliefs and not necessarily the tenets of a recognized organized religion. Most states, including Illinois, have adopted the definition of personal as decided by Judge Wexler in a New York case.

> Until 1987 New York's law requiring vaccination of school-aged children provided a religious exemption only to "bona fide members of a recognized religious organization," but in that year a United States district judge ruled that limiting the exemption in this manner was unconstitutional.

The United States Constitution mandates that, if New York wishes to allow a religiously-based exclusion from its otherwise compulsory program of immunization of school children, it may not limit this exception from the program to members of specific religious groups, but must offer the exemption to all persons who sincerely hold religious beliefs that prohibit the inoculation of their children by the state.

Judge Leonard D. Wexler
United States District Court, Eastern District of New York
October 21, 1987

As a result of the decision New York amended its law to read:

This section shall not apply to children whose parent, parents, or guardian hold genuine and sincere religious beliefs which are contrary to the practices herein required, and no certificate shall be required as a prerequisite to such children being admitted or received into school or attending school.

Illinois law §665.510 also states that

> "The local school authority is responsible
> for determining whether the written
> statement constitutes a valid religious
> objection".

At the present time there is no Illinois case law
interpreting this element of the statute. Therefore one
can look to other state law for interpretation. Even
though other state law would not be binding for the
state of Illinois, it would be very influential in judicial
settings where Illinois case law does not address the
issue. In May 2001 the Wyoming Supreme Court in
<u>Susan LePage vs. The State of Wyoming Department of
Health</u> ruled on this very issue.

> [¶15] We do not believe that the legislature,
> through its adoption of §21 -4-309(a),
> anticipated or authorized a broad
> investigation into an individual's belief
> system in an effort to discern the merit of
> a request for exemption. Rather, we
> construe the statutory language as
> mandatory and the exemption as self-
> executing upon submission of a written
> objection.

(For a fuller version of the opinion see Appendix C
page 1.)

Illinois courts would most probably hold that the
presenting in writing of a personal religious objection
to vaccinations stating the specific religious reasons for
the objection would be self executing (would be
automatically accepted). Therefore, as in the findings of
the Wyoming Supreme Court, Illinois courts would
most probably find that if the school board tries to
assess the sincerity of one's religious conviction it
would be a First Amendment freedom of religion issue.

Remedies

The National Institute of Health (NIH) should call for a consensus conference of 20 - 25 of the top scientists in the country. These scientists will evaluate the scientific literature with regard to childhood vaccines both pro and con. Then they will produce a consensus statement. This consensus statement would reflect a more accurate scientific assessment of the literature on childhood vaccinations.

When these consensus committees met in the past, the following conclusions were formulated:

1) Routine prenatal ultra sounds are only expensive baby pictures.
2) They found no scientific evidence that screening mammography between ages 40 and 50 increased longevity.
3) The Cesarean section rate in this country should be less than 15% - not 20-25%.

A consensus committee on vaccines would most probably come to some wise decisions to help us decide should we or should we not give vaccines to our children.

APPENDIX A
Excerpts from Illinois Compiled Statute, as well as Illinois Administrative Law

ILLINOIS COMPILED STATUTES (ILCS)

(410 ILCS 315/0.01)
Sec. 0.01. Short title. This Act may be cited as the
Communicable Disease Prevention Act.

(410 ILCS 315/1)
Sec. 1.
Certain communicable diseases such as measles, poliomyelitis and tetanus, may and do result in serious physical and mental disability including mental retardation, permanent paralysis, encephalitis, convulsions, pneumonia, and not infrequently, death.

Most of these diseases attack young children, and if they have not been immunized, may spread to other susceptible children and possibly, adults, thus, posing serious threats to the health of the community. Effective, safe and widely used vaccines and immunization procedures have been developed and are available to prevent these diseases and to limit their spread. Even though such immunization procedures are available, many children fail to receive this protection either through parental oversight, lack of concern, knowledge or interest, or lack of available facilities or funds. The existence of susceptible children in the community constitutes a health hazard to the individual and to the public at large by serving as a focus for the spread of these communicable diseases.

It is declared to be the public policy of this State that all children shall be protected, as soon after birth as medically indicated, by the appropriate vaccines and immunizing procedures to prevent communicable diseases which are or which may in the future become preventable by immunization.

(410 ILCS 315/2)
Sec. 2. **The Department of Public Health shall promulgate rules and regulations requiring immunization of children against preventable communicable diseases designated by the Director.** Before any regulation or amendment thereto is prescribed, the Department shall conduct a public hearing regarding such regulation. In addition, before any regulation or any amendment to a regulation is adopted, and after the Immunization Advisory Committee has made its recommendations, the State Board of Health shall conduct 3 public hearings, geographically distributed throughout the State, regarding the regulation or amendment to the

regulation. At the conclusion of the hearings, the State Board of Health shall issue a report, including its recommendations, to the Director. The Director shall take into consideration any comments or recommendations made by the Board based on these hearings. **The Department may prescribe additional rules and regulations for immunization of other diseases as vaccines are developed.**

The provisions of this Act shall not apply if:
1. **The parent or guardian of the child objects thereto on the grounds that the administration of immunizing agents conflicts with his religious tenets or practices or,**
2. A physician employed by the parent or guardian to provide care and treatment to the child states that the physical condition of the child is such that the administration of one or more of the required immunizing agents would be detrimental to the health of the child.

(410 ILCS 235/3)
Sec. 3. Public pamphlet. The Director shall prepare and make available upon request to all health care providers, parents and guardians in the State, a pamphlet which explains the benefits and possible

adverse reactions to immunizations for pertussis. This pamphlet may contain any information which the Director deems necessary and may be revised by the Department whenever new information concerning these immunizations becomes available. The pamphlet shall include the following information:

(a) A list of the immunizations required for admission to a public or private school in the State;

(b) Specific information regarding the pertussis vaccine which includes:

    (1) The circumstances under which pertussis vaccine should not be administered or should be delayed, including the categories of persons who are significantly more vulnerable to major adverse reactions than are members of the general population;

    (2) The frequency, severity and potential long-term effects of pertussis;

    (3) Possible adverse reactions to pertussis vaccine and the early warning signs or symptoms that may be precursors to a major adverse reaction which, upon occurrence, should be brought to the immediate attention of the health care provider who administered the vaccine;

(4) A form that the parent or guardian may use to monitor symptoms of a possible adverse reaction and which includes places where the parent or guardian can record information about the symptoms that will assist the health care provider; and

(5) Measures that a parent or guardian should take to reduce the risk of, or to respond to, a maj or adverse reaction including identification of who should be notified of the reaction and when the notification should be made.

The Director shall prepare the pamphlet in consultation with the Illinois State Medical Society, the Illinois Hospital Association, and interested consumer groups and shall adopt by regulation the information contained in the pamphlet, pursuant to the Administrative Procedure Act.

77 ILLINOIS ADMINISTRATIVE CODE
TITLE 77: PUBLIC HEALTH
PART 665
CHILD HEALTH EXAMINATION CODE

K-12 School Immunization Requirements

Section 665.100 Statutory **Authority**

The Illinois Department of Public Health
(Department) is authorized under Section
27-8.1 of the School Code (Ill. Rev. Stat.
1991. Ch. 122. Par. 27-8.1) *[105* ILCS
5/27-8.1] TO PROMULGATE THE RULES
AND REGULATIONS, SPECIFY THE
EXAMINATIONS AND PROCEDURES
WHICH SHALL CONSTITUTE A HEALTH
EXAMINATION, AND TO PROMULGATE
RULES AND REGULATIONS SPECIFYING
IMMUNIZATIONS AGAINST
PREVENTABLE COMMUNICABLE
DISEASES.

Section 665.230 School Entrance

a) Every child, prior to enrolling in any
public, private/independent or

parochial school (includes nursery schools, pre-school programs, early childhood programs, Head Start, or other pre-kindergarten child care programs offered or operated by a school or school district) in Illinois shall present to that school proof of immunity against:

1) Diphtheria

2) Pertussis

3) Tetanus

4) Poliomyelitis

5) Measles

6) Rubella

7) Mumps

8) Haemophilus influenzae type B

9) Hepatitis B

(Chicken Pox Vaccine as of May 2002)

Section 665.270 Compliance with the Law

A child shall be considered in compliance with the law if all immunizations which a child can medically receive are given prior to entering school and a signed statement from a health care provider is presented indicated when the remaining medically indicated immunization will be received. Immunization schedules must be monitored by local school authorities to assure completion of the immunization schedule. If a child is delinquent for a scheduled appointment for immunization he/she is no longer considered in compliance.

Section 665.280 Physician Statement of Immunity

A physician licensed to practice medicine in all of its branches, who believes a child to be protected against a disease for which immunization is required may so indicate in writing, stating the reasons, and certify that he/she believes the specific immunization in question is not necessary or indicated. Such a statement should be attached to the child's school health record and accepted as satisfying the medical exception provision of the regulation for that immunization. **These statements of lack of medical need will be reviewed by the Department with appropriate medical consultation.** After review, if a student is no longer considered to be in compliance, the student is subject to the exclusion provision of the law.

Section 665.510 Objection **of Parent or Legal Guardian**

Parent or legal guardian of a student may object to health examinations, immunizations, vision and hearing screening tests, and dental health examination for their children on religious grounds. If a religious objection is made, a written and signed statement from the parent or legal guardian detailing such objections must be presented to the local school authority. The objection must set forth the specific religious belief which conflicts with the examination, immunization or other medical intervention. **The religious objection may be personal and need not be directed by the tenets of an established religious organization.** General philosophical or moral reluctance to allow physical examinations, immunizations, vision and hearing screening, and dental examinations will not provide a sufficient basis for an exception to statutory requirements. **The local school authority is responsible for determining whether the written statement constitutes a valid religious objection.** The parent or legal guardian must be informed by the local school authority of measles outbreak control exclusion procedures in accordance with the Department's rules, Control of Communicable

Appendix A

Diseases Code (77 Ill. Adm. Code 690) at the time such objection is presented.

Section 665.520 Medical Objection

a) Any medical objection to an immunization must be:

1) Made by a physician licensed to practice medicine in all its branches indicating what the medical condition is.

2) Endorsed and signed by physician on the certificate of child health examination and placed on file in the child's permanent record.

b) Should the condition of the child later permit immunization, this requirement will then have to be met. Parents or legal guardians must be informed of measles outbreak control exclusion procedures when such objection is presented per Section 665.510.

APPENDIX B
Illinois Law with Regard to
Newborn Vaccine Mandates

Most Illinois hospitals administer the hepatitis B vaccine within 24 hours of birth. Ms. Eaton, a member of the Illinois Immunization Advisory Committee, questioned the IDPH if this is an Illinois law, or are hospitals and doctors doing this on their own.

To:　RICHARD GALATI [RGALATI@idph.state.il.us]
　　　Illinois Department of Public Health

Sent:　Monday, August 27, 2001

From:　Fran Eaton
　　　Eagle Forum of Illinois

Subject:　Illinois Law with Regard to Newborn
　　　Vaccine Mandates

Could you tell me where in Illinois law it states that all newborns are required to receive the hepatitis B immunization [within 24 hours after birth]? I understand it is a requirement for admission to day care, but where is the law requiring its administration for newborns?

Thanks for any help you can give.

Fran Eaton

<u>**REPLY**</u>

To: Fran Eaton
            Eagle Forum of Illinois

Sent: Monday, August 27, 2001

From: RICHARD GALATI [RGALATI@idph.state.il.us]
            Illinois Department of Public Health

Subject: Re: Reference in Illinois Code

There is no state statute REQUIRING newborns to be vaccinated against any vaccine-preventable disease, including hepatitis B. It is the only currently licensed vaccine that can be given to infants shortly after birth. The other recommended vaccines (such as DTaP, Polio, Hib and Pneumococcal conjugate) are not recommended for administration until the infant is 6 weeks of age or older (i.e. on or about 2 months of age). **The immunization rules require children two years of age and older enrolled in child care facilities to be immunized against hepatitis B.** Hope this answers your question.

M.E. Comments

The above response from the Illinois Department of Public Health rules that the Illinois mandates for Hepatitis B Vaccine does not become effective until two years of age unless your child is enrolled in day care or preschool. Administration of Hepatitis B Vaccine by hospitals within 24 hours of birth is their medical decision, not the state law.

APPENDIX C
Vaccination Legislation SB 1305
in Illinois Becomes Illinois Law October 2001

SB 1305 (Illinois Senate Bill 1305 Amends the Juvenile Court Act of 1987 and Adoption Act) Removes **"not immunizing"** as reason for investigation by [Illinois] Department of Children and Family Services (DCFS)

> **"A child shall not be considered neglected or abused for the sole reason that the child's parent or other person responsible for the child's welfare failed to vaccinate, delayed vaccination, or refused vaccination for the child whether due to a waiver on religious or medical grounds as permitted by the law."**

Based on SB1305 the IDCFS promulgated the following change to Administrative Rule 300 which was approved by The Joint Committee on Administrative Rules (JCAR*) effective October 1, 2001.

Allegation #79 - Medical Neglect - has had all references to immunizations removed. Therefore,

> **we will no longer be accepting reports on situations where a lack of**

immunizations is the only allegation.
State Central Registry (SCR) staff
should refer reporters to the
Department of Public Health. Child
Protection Investigators (CPs) who are
currently investigating reports where a
lack of immunizations is the only
allegation should "Initially Unfound"
them if they are still within the 14 day
time frame. If not, supervisors should
review the reports and waive additional
contacts so they can be Unfounded.
Exceptions should be made if the
investigation has revealed other
potential harms.

**Two purposes of the committee are to ensure that the
Legislature is adequately informed of how laws are
implemented through agency rulemaking and to facilitate
public understanding of rules and regulations.** To that end, in
addition to the review of new and existing rulemaking, the
committee monitors legislation that affects rulemaking and
conducts a public act review to alert agencies to the need for
rulemaking....

Illinois Blue Book
1997-1998
Page 134

M.E. Comments

SB 1305 removes IDCFS' regulation of medical neglect for parents who choose to delay vaccination, fail or refuse to vaccinate their children based on medical or religious exemptions. This was adopted by the Illinois Department of Children and Family Services' [IDCFS] and approved by JCAR*

As determined in the House floor debate, SB 1305's legislative intent, also, includes families who delay or refuse vaccination for their children's developmental problems, e.g., Down Syndrome or minor illnesses.

With SB 1305, doctors are free to advocate different vaccination schedules than recommended by medical societies for developmental issues or minor illnesses without writing a medical exemption.

*JCAR –The Joint Committee on Administrative Rules is a bipartisan legislative oversight committee created by the General Assembly in 1977. Pursuant to the Illinois Administrative Procedure Act, the committee is authorized to conduct systematic reviews of administrative rules promulgated by state agencies. The committee conducts several integrated review programs, including a review program for proposed, emergency and peremptory rulemaking, a review of new public acts and a complaint review program.

The committee is composed of 12 legislators who are appointed by the legislative leadership, and the membership is apportioned equally between the two houses and the two political parties. Members serve two-year terms, and the committee is co-chaired by a member of each party and legislative house. Support services for the committee are provided by 25 staff members.

APPENDIX D

IN THE SUPREME COURT, STATE OF WYOMING

2110 WY 26 - March 8, 2001

OCTOBER TERM, A.D. 2000

Excerpts from Susan LePage vs. State of Wyoming, Department of Health

...The statute provides mandatory language, and the Department of Health may not circumvent the legislature's clear limitation of its powers or expand its power beyond its statutory authority. There is no justification found within the statute for the Department of Health to institute a religious inquiry. As a result, the decision to do so is not in accordance with the law.

[¶ 14] Furthermore, construing the statute as the Department of Health suggests raises questions concerning the extent to which the government should be involved in the religious lives of its citizens. Should an individual be forced to present evidence of his/her religious beliefs to be scrutinized by a governmental employee? If parents have not consistently expressed those religious beliefs over time, should they be denied an exemption? Can parents have beliefs that are both philosophical and religious without disqualifying their exemption request? Should the government require a certain level of sincerity as a benchmark before an exemption can be granted? If the legislature chose to address these types of questions with further legislation, such legislation would call into question the constitutional prohibition against governmental interference with the free exercise of religion under Article 1, Section 18 of the Wyoming Constitution. However, those issues need not be addressed in this case because the statute does not provide the authority for such inquiry.

[¶15] We do not believe that the legislature, through its adoption of § 21 -4-309(a), anticipated or authorized a broad investigation into an individual's belief system in an effort to discern the merit of a request for exemption. Rather, we construe the statutory language as mandatory and the exemption as self-executing upon submission of a written objection.

[¶16] In her request for exemption, Mrs. LePage fully complied with both the statutory and the regulatory requirements. However, it should be noted that, in attempting to enforce the immunization for hepatitis B, the Department of Health failed to abide by its own regulations which do not include the hepatitis B vaccination. Department of Health Rules, *Immunization Regulations,* ch. 1, § 7(b) (1-13-92). "An administrative agency must follow its own rules and regulations." *Antelope Valley Improvement v. State Board of Equalization for State of Wyoming,* 992 P.2d 563, 566 (Wyo. 1999), *opinion clarified at* 4 P.3d 876 (Wyo. 2000). This could be an independent reason for reversing the State Health Officer's conclusion that a religious waiver was necessary for exemption from the hepatitis B vaccination.

[¶17] **We recognize the genuine concern that there could be increased requests for exemption and a potential for improper evasion of immunization. The state certainly has a valid interest in protecting public schoolchildren from unwarranted exposure to infectious diseases. However, we have been presented with no evidence that the number of religious exemption waiver requests are excessive** and are confident in our presumption that parents act in the best interest of their children's physical, as well as their spiritual, health. Again, if problems regarding the health of Wyoming's schoolchildren develop because this self-executing statutory exemption is being abused, it is the legislature's responsibility to act within the constraints of the Wyoming and United States Constitutions.

Appendix E

Elements of an Illinois Religious Exemption Letter Concerning Mandated Childhood Vaccines

Following is an outline of a religious waiver letter regarding childhood vaccines. It is meant as a reference to point out the necessary and required elements as defined by Illinois law. It is not meant as a form letter. Each family must assess their religious beliefs or the tenets of their church to see if they meet the requirements of a valid religious exemption.

1) Dear local school authority...

2) We are the parents/legal guardian of...

3) We are exercising our rights as Illinois citizens...

4) Under Illinois Administrative Code § 665.510...
   (page 157)[10]

5) (a)   We are setting forth our **specific** religious
         personal objection why our religious beliefs

---

[10] You should quote the Administrative Code §665.510 verbatim.

are in conflict with giving childhood vaccinations...[11]

or,

(b) we are setting forth our specific religious objections based on the **tenets** of our established religious organization.[12]

---

[11] You must set forth specific religious beliefs, i.e. passages from scripture. The specific personal religious objection cannot be medical, i.e., vaccines are dangerous therefore I religiously object. Since the scientific literature has articles pro and con with regard to childhood vaccines, it would be difficult to make scientific evidence based decision based on the medical literature. Therefore, if you are a religious person, the reason you would be objecting would most probably be religious not medical. i.e. I don't believe God allows human beings to inject foreign substances into their bodies. If your objection mentions anything medical, it becomes a medical exemption, (must be written by a licensed Illinois physician as discussed in 141), not a personal religious exemption.

[12] To be in compliance with the law you need to select (a) or (b), you do not need both.)

6) Both parents should sign the letter in front of a notary.[13]

---

[13] This is not a legal requirement, however, in case of divorce or separation one spouse could not claim that he or she was against not vaccinating without recanting the original religious position.

APPENDIX F

BIBLICAL & RELIGIOUS REFERENCES

"We believe in God, and that God has created us in his image. In being created in God's image, we are given his perfect immune system. We are bestowed with His gift, the immune system. We believe it is sacrilegious and a violation of our sacred religious beliefs to violate what God has given us by showing a lack of faith in God. Immunizations are a lack of faith in God and His way, the immune system."

"We believe in Jesus' many promises of protection for us, and the He loves us, and will take care of us if we place our trust in Him. I believe that immunizations show no faith in God's promises of protection for us, saying to God that you trust man more than His holy words of protection for us."

"God desires us to love Him and our neighbors first and foremost. This is His first command. By loving Him, we are to fully trust on Him for all things. He is our Lord Father. He is our Rock, our fortress and our Savior."

"Our faith is in God and in the Holy Word, being the Holy Bible which is authored by God. This is the instruction book for living that He has left us and in it

He tells us He is our protector and we stand firm on His promise. Our faith is in Him!"

"And hearing this, Jesus said to them, 'It is not those who are healthy who need a physician, but those who are sick; I did not come to call the righteous, but sinners.'" (Mark 2:17)

"Know ye not that your body is the temple of the Holy Ghost which is in you, which ye have of God and ye are not your own?" (1st COR 6:19)

"That your faith should not stand in the wisdom of men, but in the power of God." (1st COR 2:5)

"You must know that your body is a temple of the Holy Spirit, who is within the spirit you have received from God. You are not your own." (1st COR 6:19)

"As a consequence, your faith rests not on the wisdom of men but on the power of God." (1st COR 2:5)

"I know with certainly on the authority of Lord Jesus that nothing is unclean in itself: it is only when a man thinks something unclean that it becomes so for him." (Romans 14:14)

"If anyone destroys God's temple, God will destroy him. For the temple of God is holy, and you are that temple."(lst COR: 3:17)

"For to his angels he has given command about you, that they guard you in all your ways." (Psalms 91:11)

"Follow God your Lord, remain in awe of him, keep His commandments, obey and serve Him and you will then be able to cling to Him." (Leviticus, 19:1,2)

Appendix G

Questions & Answers with Regard

To Childhood Vaccines

Q) Are vaccine mandates federal or state?

A) All vaccine legislation at the present time is state law not federal law.

Q) What is a philosophical objection to vaccines?

A) A philosophical objection to vaccines states that you are objecting from your own personal belief, not on medical or religious grounds. It comes from your own personal knowledge whatever that is composed of. At the time of this writing Illinois does not accept this as a valid objection to childhood vaccines. A philosophical objection is also known as a constitutional objection, (as defined by the *American College Dictionary* - belonging to or inherent in a person's constitution of body or mind) not to be confused with the U.S. Constitution.

Q) What is a medical exemption to vaccines?

A) An exemption that is written by a physician who is licensed to practice in the state stating the specific medical objections to the vaccine.

Q) What are state mandates?

A) Childhood vaccine rules and regulations are promulgated by each state. Therefore, each state can determine which vaccines are required for your child's protection. The list of required vaccines can vary from state to state. These required vaccines are called mandates. At present, Illinois mandates DPT, MMR, HIB, Polio, Hepatitis B, and Chicken Pox Vaccines.

Q) Do vaccines weaken the immune system?

A) The scientific literature has mixed reviews. Some studies say yes (see page 1) Some scientific studies say no (see page 23)

Q) Can I give some of the vaccines and not others?

A) Yes, from a medical standpoint. However, to be in compliance with the state laws you must give your children the mandated vaccines unless you have a religious, philosophical or medical waiver exemption. You must check your state's law to see which of the waiver exemptions apply. Illinois only considers medical or religious waivers.

Q) What is SV40?

A) SV40 stands for Simian (monkey) virus #40. SV 40 was a contaminant in the polio vaccines given between 1953 and 1963. See page 42. It was the 40th Simian virus discovered as a contaminant in the polio vaccine. What makes SV40 so critical is that it has been implicated in human cancers and has been transmitted to children from their parents via genetic material.

Q) Which vaccines are mandated in Illinois?

A) DPT, MMR, HIB, Polio, Hepatitis B, and Chicken Pox Vaccines.

Q) Are there medical contraindications to vaccines?

A) It depends which side of the debate you are on. Scientific medical studies seem to point in both directions - that there are benefits and side effects. The difficulty is deciding which are more controlling.

Q) Can I give some of the mandated vaccines and not the others?

A) Not if you want to be in compliance with the law. Unless you have a medical, religious, or philosophical exemption, i.e. you may object to the Chicken Pox Vaccine merely on the basis that it was grown on the cells of aborted fetuses, but not object to the other vaccines.

Q) What is a personal religious exemption?

A) It is an exemption that states your personal religious beliefs. These beliefs may not necessarily be the tenets or beliefs of you established or organized religion.

Q) If I homeschool my children do I have to give childhood vaccines?

A) Yes, the mandate for vaccines has nothing to do with school. School is just a checkpoint to see if you have given the mandated vaccines. A response from the Illinois Department of Public Health says that no vaccine mandates are in effect under two years of age (see page 160), unless you enroll your child (under the age of two) in pre-school or day care.

Q) At what age does the vaccine mandate take effect?

A) See previous question.

Q) Can I be reported to DCFS (Department of Child and Family Services) if I do not vaccinate?

A) Yes. Unless you have a bonafide exemption medical or religious (and in some states philosophical). If your child is less than two years of age and not in pre-school or day care, the mandates do not apply. (See page 160)

Q) What are specific religious grounds objecting to vaccines?

A) They are statements which bring out your religious beliefs and religious reasons for objecting to childhood vaccines. These statements can come from the Bible, the tenets of your established religion, or your personal religious beliefs.

Q) If I use a religious exemption does it have to be signed by a clergyman?

A) No. Illinois courts have held that a religious exemption does not have to be on church stationary, does not have to be signed by a clergyman and does not necessarily have to be the tenets of your church.

Q) Can the state decide if your religious exemption is valid?

A) Illinois has a statute which allows the School Board to determine the sincerity of your religious belief. (See page 157) There are no Illinois cases which address the constitutionality of this statute. If challenged in court, even though it would not be precedent setting, the courts would look for guidance to other states ruling on similar statutes. Based on a Wyoming Supreme Court Case, (see page 167) if challenged in court, Illinois courts would find the Illinois statute allowing the school board to determine the validity and sincerity of your personal religious beliefs to be in violation of First Amendment rights.

Q) Can the state review your personal physician's letter objection to vaccines on medical grounds?

A) Yes. The state has the right to appoint another physician or consultant to review your physician's medical exemption. The courts would probably find this to be a valid and constitutional. (See page 156.)

Q) Are any of the vaccines good?

A) Scientific studies exist on both sides of the issue. Mandates aside, at this time there is no clear cut answer.

Q) Which vaccines should I give?

A) That becomes again a difficult question to answer for the same reason as given above.

Q) If vaccines really work, why should other children who are vaccinated worry?

A) That is a good question. I suppose that the vaccine proponents don't have as much faith in these vaccines as they would like us to believe.

Q) Do the vaccines work or are the diseases no longer around?

A) That goes to the heart of the statistical scientific debate. Some diseases like plague, tuberculosis, etc. were widespread and even without the use of vaccines just seemed to die out.

Q) What other substances are in vaccines?

A) See partial list on page xiv.

Q) Is hepatitis B a sexually transmitted disease?

A) Yes. See the Center for Disease Control recommendation who is at risk for hepatitis B on page 1.

Q) Is the Chicken Pox Vaccine grown on the cells of aborted fetuses?

A) Yes. The Chicken Pox Vaccine is grown on a culture of diploid tissue. Diploid is defined as human tissue. The Chicken Pox Vaccine is grown on the cells of aborted fetuses. The original culture has been replicated over and over again so is does not require new fetuses to be aborted for the production of the vaccine. However, one who receives the Chicken Pox Vaccine is directly linked to the chain that goes back to the original abortion.

Q) Is the rubella vaccine gown on the cells of aborted fetuses?

A) Yes. See above answer.

Q) Is the MMR vaccine linked to autism?

A) Some studies say yes, some studies say no. At the present time there is no conclusive, definitive scientific evidence.

Q) Is mercury still in vaccines?

A) Yes. It is still in the flu vaccine which is now being recommended to our children (see page 22).

Q) Can I object to only Chicken Pox Vaccine on religious grounds, because I am pro-life, without objecting to any other vaccines?

A) Yes, if your religious convictions are pro life and you object to the Chicken Pox Vaccine because it was grown on the cells of aborted fetuses. However, like all waivers, medical or religious, it could be challenged by the school board. The Illinois courts would most probably uphold this waiver as a valid religious exemption, see page167.

Q) Do physicians respect parents' rights to debate issues of vaccines?

A) They should, however, most physicians would respond to that question like Dr. Ben Katz from Childrens Memorial Hospital (April 11th, 2002 issue of "Daily Southtown") "We need to force people to do right thing [vaccine], unfortunately. We can't leave these decisions up to individuals. I really believe it is inappropriate to debate this with parents."

EPILOGUE

Falsus in uno, falsus in
omnibus. Untrue in one thing,
untrue in everything.

Latin Expression

20th Century medicine has been shown to be false in many of its assumptions and it has held physicians with non-interventionist philosophies to a higher standard than interventionist physicians. The unscientific thinking of "I think therefore I believe" has replaced scientific evidence based decision making. How can we have trust in a medical system which has been shown to be untrue in some of its practice? The answer is with great scepticism. Let us pray that scientific reason will prevail and the motto for the 21st Century will become **"The scientific evidence points in that direction, therefore I believe"**.

INDEX

About Homefirst®

Homefirst® Health Services provides a full range of services in family health care in the greater Chicago metropolitan area with six medical centers - 847/679-8336 or www.homefirst.com. Our group of doctors, nurses, and certified nurse midwives dedicate themselves to providing the highest quality of health care while maintaining personalized care for each patient and family. We encourage patient involvement in the many decisions made regarding their health care.

Our care begins many times before life itself. Many couples will come to Homefirst® for pre-conception counseling. We encourage health habits that maximize the greatest chance in conceiving, maintaining a healthy pregnancy, and giving birth with the greatest efficiency and personal reward. We promote the most natural way to labor and give birth, thus avoiding unnecessary medical interventions and where the goal of an uncomplicated delivery is most likely to occur. In addition, we offer state of the art obstetrical and neonatal care if the situation calls for it. This obstetrical system has attained the highest rates of successful vaginal births and has shown that women can safely give birth at home and reap the many benefits in doing so, including a joyful and rewarding experience.

The care of the family continues after the baby is born. Breastfeeding is promoted as the foundation to maintaining the health of the newborn. It is unsurpassed in giving the baby proper nutrition. In addition, mother's milk is a source of countless other health benefits including prevention of respiratory infections, gastrointestinal illness, metabolic illness and allergies. Breast milk also contains neuropeptides which have been shown to promote brain development. Because of these advantages, Homefirst® has many resources to support the nursing relationship. Many of our nurses and receptionists are LaLeche League leaders. We also have certified lactation consultants to address the more challenging and technical problems the mother may experience.

Homefirst® also provides a full range of pediatric services as well as women's and men's health care. We continue to emphasize the philosophy of minimal use of drugs and surgery and maximal patient involvement in maintaining good health for everyone. We promote an integrative evidence based approach to managing illness. The majority of health problems are taken care of by our medical staff. When necessary, we provide referrals to a wide variety of consultants which include practitioners in alternative approaches to medicine as well as conventional medical specialists.

It has been an honor and a privilege to serve families for over 30 years, to deliver more than 15,000 babies at home and serve over 75,000 mothers, fathers, children and extended family members. Our greatest pleasure has been to provide the opportunity for our patients to grow and enrich their lives with the knowledge they are taking charge over their own health and maximizing their greatest health potential.

About the Author
Dr. Mayer Eisenstein

Dr. Mayer Eisenstein is a graduate of the University of Illinois Medical School, the Medical College of Wisconsin School of Public Health, and the John Marshall Law School.

Since 1973 he has been in private medical practice and is currently the Medical Director of Homefirst® Health Services, the largest physician attended home birth service in the country. In his 30 years in medicine, he and his practice have delivered over 15,000 babies at home, as well as cared for over 75,000 parents, grandparents and children. Now, Dr. Eisenstein and his practice are delivering second generation babies for women who themselves were born at home with his practice.

He is Board Certified by the National Board of Medical Examiners, American Board of Public Health and Preventive Medicine, and the American Board of Quality Assurance and Utilization Review Physicians. He is a member of the National Honor Society. He is a recipient of the Howard Fellowship, Health Professional Scholarship, University of Illinois School of Medicine Scholarship, and is a member of the Illinois Bar.

He is on the Professional Board of the Family Life League, Council for the Jewish Elderly, Task Force Council on Education for Public Health - Medical College of Wisconsin, and on the Editorial Board for "Child and Family Magazine". He is the author of the award winning book *Give Birth at Home With The Home Birth Advantage*, and *Safer Medicine*. His medical film "Primum Non Nocere" (Above All Do No Harm), a documentary on home birth, was an award winner at the Chicago Film Festival in 1987.

Some of his guest appearances include: the "Phil Donahue Show", "Milt Rosenberg Show", "Today in Chicago", "Ask the Expert", "Daybreak", "Oprah Winfrey Show", "Ed Schwartz Radio Show". "WMAQ TV news 'Unnecessary Hysterectomy'", "Chicago Fox TV News - 'Immunizations - Are They Necessary'", CBC Newsworld Canada - "Are Mass Immunizations Necessary".

Since 1987, his weekly radio show "Family Health Forum", has aired in the Chicagoland area. In the live call-in format, all listener's comments, questions or medical experiences are welcome by Dr. Eisenstein.

Dr. Eisenstein's philosophy comes from his years in medicine, combined with his years as a husband, father, and grandfather (he has six children and six grandchildren).

Notes

Notes